The Body's Emotional Imprint

Thea Maii

Disclaimer: The content of this book is for informational purposes only and is in no way intended as a substitute for qualified medical intervention. Nor is the information intended to provide medical advice, or prevent, cure or diagnose illness.

ISNB # 978-0-9845118-5-3

Cover and interior design: Jim Bisakowski, www.BookDesign.ca

For Magnus and Phoebe

Also by Thea Maii

The Emotional Imprint of Clutter

Contents

A — Z

Systems of the Body

Circulatory

      Heart   Blood

Respiratory

      Lungs   Nose

Digestive

Mouth	Jaw	Stomach
Liver	Gall Bladder	Pancreas
Small Intestine	Colon	Bowel

Urinary

      Kidney   Bladder

Reproductive

      Breasts   Genitals Ovaries

      Prostate

Endocrine

      Adrenals   Thyroid Pineal

      Pituitary

Immune

      Lymphatic system   Spleen

Musculoskeletal

Chest	Shoulders	Arms
Wrist	Hand	Hips
Knees	Ankles	Spine
Legs	Feet	

Nervous

Spinal Cord	Brain	Head
Ears	Eyes	Neck

Skin

      Bruises   Cuts

Introduction

Good health, most of us were brought up to believe, would be the reward for leading a healthy lifestyle incorporating good food, exercise and charitable thoughts. The rules were always a little vague, though, about what constituted good food, leaving us to be a little vague with them as we looked at the pyramid picture the government put out telling us what to eat and in what quantities. But just how big is a serving of vegetables, and who's appetite is it based on? We know that technically a tomato is a fruit but we eat it as a vegetable, so which column do we put it in? Are the figures based on one large potato or one small? And how do you count calories without a chart?

And so, as with most things in our lives that take time to comprehend, we have based our eating habits more on instant gratification than on future health benefits. Now, after years of being bombarded with research figures and experts extolling the virtues of this or that diet, we are beginning to understand that our bodies are not the simple machines we all thought they were, but are in fact a complex array of cells, minerals, electrical impulses, and a whole host of other things that form one carefully constructed unit. And the more information we have uncovered, the more many of us have turned to alternative medicine to make sense of the whole human design.

As the world opened up to us in the 1960's, with easier travel and a yearning to explore other countries and cultures, so a cross pollination of ideas also took root, with religion, foods and medicine all crossing over onto a pathway that has over the past few decades taken many twists and turns, connecting us back to our natural heritage, other cultures and our own intuitive knowledge in search of less invasive and more comprehensive ways to know both the body and the mind.

As we've muddled through the process of how the body interacts with everything that it takes in—pharmaceutical drugs, pollutants, pesticides and all manner of toxins and chemicals—information overload has also kicked in, leaving us rushing from one extreme to the other as each new piece of information seems to supersede the one before. We know what the end result should be, but how do we get there? If sperm count is down in industrialized nations, as research seems to bear out, then obviously other cells must be dying too, including, and maybe especially, cells that are important to our future health and well-being and to a fully functional biological system.

Only now are we beginning to understand through Epigenetics—defined as a heritable influence on gene expression that does not involve changes to the underlying DNA sequence—that chemical markers can be passed on from previous generations to future ones, even if offspring are never exposed to the original substance. As this accumulative effect continues, so too does the damage caused by the accumulation, which may be a large reason for the explosion of Autism and other illnesses. From the 1950's onwards, each successive generation has been exposed to an ever increasing amount of vaccinations, pesticides and all manner of chemicals that have been added to the food and water supply.

As our understanding has increased on how foods, toxins and emotions are passed on from the mother to the fetus, so the whole birth process should now be in question—along with just how much medical intervention we should allow into our own and our children's lives. In Western culture, birth is now relegated to a process that accommodates the doctor rather than the mother and child's psychological well-being. We give birth in sterile surroundings, under bright fluorescent lights, with the mother in a position not conducive to pushing the baby out, in a room full of strangers—often with surgical instruments pulling at the baby's head—and drugs pumped into our bodies. And from this we expect calm, emotionally nourished, intelligent children to emerge. Given our over-medicated, obese, learning disabled, hyper children, obviously nothing could be further from the truth.

Good health, however, has as much to do with emotional stability as physical dexterity, and not being able to use our true intellectual capacity can lead to illness as much as a bad diet, disease or poverty. How much control we are able to exert over our lives from childhood on, is usually expressed in the level of health we achieve throughout our lives, with lack of control often turning into depression, fear, anger, withdrawal, or an inability to concentrate. In other words, who we become is a representation of both our emotional and physical world, with illness springing up where emotions have been closed down. The words we use, the colors we dislike, the sounds we gravitate to, the fluidity of our movements, the lines and shape of our faces, palms and eyes, all indicate the path we have consciously, unconsciously and subconsciously followed.

How balanced our lives are is also indicated by how balanced our bodies and minds are, and yet while balance in the East is something to strive towards, in the West it has always represented a state of boredom, excitement being the order of the day. And part of our inability to accept quietude and be one with nature comes from being taught at an early age that we should be in constant motion, constantly doing some activity, and that time is money. Children's lives are now so full of extracurricular activities that there is little time to play alone quietly, which in all probability, is part of the reason for the increase in Attention Deficit Disorder. But how much of that filling up space and time is really for the benefit of parents who no longer know how to just "be" with their children, and who are themselves overloaded, constantly on the move and constantly striving to accumulate more?

Over the centuries, too, our balance has also been thrown off by taking sides according to which hemisphere of the brain we predominantly work from, with our educational system geared to left-brain predominance and away from a whole-brain system, and with the arts, sports and creativity dispensed with at each cut in school funding. People exclaim with pride that they are a right -or left-brain-thinker, as if one foot is constantly nailed to the floor and they see only out of one eye. But one hemisphere's predominance eventually leads to a one-sided view on life, which over time distorts our body, mind and world view and is the basis for many of our global ills today as it produces a limited view of both ourselves and those who are different.

Miss any of the steps in our emotional development, from birth onwards, and it shortcut the circuits, leaving the emotions pushing and pulling our bodies and minds into contortions they were never made to make. And once we fully understand the whole-body connection to our illnesses, then medicine of the future will take on a very different form. As we see the solutions to our energy crisis lying in the hands of nature, so we also see the solutions to our well-being in those same hands, the ones we relied on for thousands of years before we put our trust into technology, chemicals and specialized medicine. Future health systems should incorporate testing for minerals, vitamins and blood type, administered at various times from birth onwards, in order to form a blueprint for any medical intervention based on the individual rather than using a one-size-fits-all method, and by documenting hand, face and eye prints at various stages of life. And health histories will record supplements, pharmaceutical drugs, illness, moods, accidents, medical intervention, X-Rays and CT scans, in order to chronicle and coordinate specific protocols for the individual. After all, if our DNA and fingerprints are all so different, then our chemical composition must also be dissimilar, something we should now take into consideration when giving vaccinations and drugs.

We are not brought up to demand a record of every doctor or hospital visit or every drug prescribed, and yet at some point the documentation could save our lives, or at least save us from other serious illnesses, and as over 100 thousand Americans die due to pharmaceutical drugs and over 2 million more suffer adverse reactions to pharmaceutical drugs each year (the numbers vary greatly according to how they are counted and who is counting), it is obviously in our best interest to start the documentation process as soon as possible. As illness can often take years or even decades to manifest, keeping all documentation will be imperative in order to chronicle our health history to see where the weakness or overload may have occurred. This is why we should do blood testing on all children before they are vaccinated so that we have a better idea of how the chemicals will interact with those already in the body. As of now, we don't collect this information before we vaccinate, but we should, and not just for children. Many elderly who are admitted to hospitals are automatically given pharmaceutical drugs, even though they may never have taken many before. Dropping an assortment of chemicals into a frail, sick body may actually be doing more harm than good, especially as many of the drugs can cause severe reactions.

The choice of how much control we exert over our health and well-being is ours to take. We can choose to see life as a glorious, exciting journey where we are the drivers, or as a slow, painful trip towards death. Knowledge is power and used wisely it can propel us into a future of less stress, more productivity and easier living—in short, more balanced lives, more intellectual freedom and greater physical ability. And as an added bonus, it will in the future, allow us to choose leaders not by their bank balances and promises but by health indicators, which gives us a much more definitive way of knowing who they truly are. Distortion in the minds of a society leads to distorted governments, economic systems and the entire workings of a culture. A society—and its political process—can only be as healthy as its citizens.

Initiation of Illness

The cement that holds every group and family together is a carefully constructed denial system that has been woven, built and patched over generations in order to get them through lives that have fallen short of childhood dreams and potential. Bonded together to shield lives lived more for neighbors and acquaintances than self-fulfillment, and where vitality has been drained by the systematic burden of disappointment, anger and finally apathetic acceptance as the years pass beneath brutal excuses that allowed them to slip away.

But as this cement weakens in our middle years, so too do our bodies and emotional equilibrium, bringing on sickness, mid-life crises and feelings of inadequacy, obsolescence and depression. The denial system that navigated us so skillfully through childhood traumas and upheavals, then becomes the very same system that trips us up in later life as the coping mechanism wears away from the overuse of steering us through turbulent lives filled with heartbreak, injustices and hurt feelings.

Family abuse, sexual, physical or verbal, often unspoken or unrecognized at the time, is endured by locking away the accompanying emotions, to be opened and dealt with at a time when the hurt has receded and the tools for coping are more sophisticated. But if that later time doesn't arrive, then the continual self-deception and false courage often leads to disease, career blocks, destructive behavior and addiction. A familiar disk of deceit replayed again and again until it dissolves into nothing more than a comforting background noise of mind-chatter.

But as the emotions dam up, so too does illness and then our sickness becomes the sickness of a society. Diseases that ravage our bodies, mirror the ravaging of the planet's resources. Our breakdowns become the breakdown of world communication, our blocked arteries, the clogged highways of the nation. Our cancers, the tumors of the political system. Our addictions, society's dependence on government, religions and the corporate world, and our obesity the bloating of those corporations. The infertility of couples mirrors the earth laid barren and heart attacks mirror the heartbreak of the pulsing planet as the life force is slowly snuffed out.

Our illnesses are the illness of a planet wallowing in excess but starved for nourishment. Too much negativity, too little caring. Too much bad behavior, too little good. Too much responsibility held by too few, not enough by the many. And as the excesses have grown, so has denial, splitting society into those willing to take responsibility for themselves and the planet, and those who won't or can't, and illness appearing within the body and the planet where the excuses congregate. Toxins in the water supply, kidney failure in the people. Nutritionally depleted soil, low functioning immune systems. Constant wars, weak adrenals. Poison dumping, colon cancer. Polluted air quality, an increase in asthma attacks. Extinction of wildlife, an increase of suicides.

Our teen years, where truth is crushed by the lies of a society and where deception features heavily, is often the genesis of our health problems, as acceptance of wrong paths taken meander into unproductive and unfulfilled lives. The untold truth, of course, is that had we been allowed to follow our bliss instead of the dictates of society, we would in later years, be happier, healthier and far more productive.

The Emotional Connection

What we think we manifest is a difficult concept for Westerners to understand, and one that had no scientific basis until the 1980's, when neuroscientists proved that mind and matter are connected, solidifying in the process that illness is as much an emotional issue as a physical one. So, which comes first? If emotional upheavals can produce physical illness, then physical illness must produce emotional ones.

The belief of much of Eastern philosophy is that we can manifest what we want by reprogramming our thought pattern and by using visualization, something many professional athletes now do and something inspirational speakers have been teaching for years. In the West we say "Be careful what you wish for" to rationalize our thought connection to an expected outcome, and say "Don't tempt fate" to ward off an unpleasant or disastrous situation. So by changing the words to more familiar ones we can understand the concept of thought producing result—except, it seems, when connecting our thoughts to health issues.

To those who catch colds each winter, it is a foregone conclusion that they always will. To those who don't, it is usually an unspoken knowledge that they won't. So mind can, and does, dictate how we respond to each situation, and how we respond emotionally can produce illness, depending on which emotion we bring to the fore.

Negative emotions such as anger, bitterness, fear, hate and self-loathing can, and do, attack a variety of organs, but love, generosity and compassion, both for ourselves and others, can also undo the damage. Just changing the words, however, doesn't banish negative emotions, which is why we have to change the molecular structure from inside as well as outside. Unfortunately, we live in a culture that is a minefield of negativity, from TV shows to the work place, and can if we allow it, override all the positive reinforcement. And Epigenetics, with the ability to change genetic expression, could presumably also include the passing of our moods and emotional composition to future generations, putting a whole different light on personality traits.

Many times our physical movement out into the world is stopped by an overprotective or overbearing parent or spouse, or self-erected obstacles that keep us downtrodden. We, on the other hand beat ourselves up as we re-circulate the words we say over and over, to the shoulders, the neck, to the arms and hands, restricting our own movement as feelings of inadequacy and fear of rejection stop us from embracing the things we really want. When we release the emotional hold then the body becomes more fluid and malleable.

Often, our thoughts precede accidents, although usually we miss the connection because of the time lapse between the emotional aspect and the physical one. People walk out of relationships well before they walk out physically, although, we nevertheless blame a third party if one is present. Broken bones can usually be traced back to fear, insecurity or a need to change direction: the snapping of our very underpinnings, a breaking away from a situation or personal involvement, a separating of one unit into two.

Accidents and sickness give us time out, time to think, time to figure out what we really want in life, in lives otherwise filled with too much noise and too many things to take care of. Accidents often happen just before some important engagement or trip. Perhaps out of fear of speaking or not wanting to have to speak in the first place. Or not wanting to take the trip alone, or with the person we are going with, or for the business we represent—or just not wanting to leave home at all.

Minor accidents happen on the way to celebrations as the mind is distracted by thoughts of what the celebration represents—marriage, birthday, family gathering—and whether it is our own or someone else's celebration. As our commitment to the event wavers, so our response may also waver— verbally, physically, or while driving a vehicle. Accidents can also be a warning that we are taking an action that is the opposite to what we truly feel we should take, perhaps by being talked into taking the action or out of obligation. We knew the deed was wrong but we did it anyway.

Illness for many, especially the elderly, can bring others into their lonely lives or it can be a form of control over the sons and daughters who left home to live their own lives. For children is can be a cry for help or attention.

Emotions can also have a profound effect on how we process foods. If we eat when we are upset or angry, it can cause the digestive system, anywhere from mouth to colon, to malfunction, and can alter the nutritional value of the substances taken in. How we look upon foods, either as friend or foe, can also alter chemical components and leave us well nourished or malnourished. Anorexics see food as the enemy and use it as a way to control others or as a cry for help. Overweight people use it for comfort. But how much of that actually comes from eating family meals in a hostile environment when young, or where food was used as a reward. Food gives life, while being an anorexic or obese can snuff it out.

We pick up on emotions at a very early age, and yet many adults talk in front of children denying that they can actually hear or comprehend. Children see and hear with clarity—before their vision is clouded by adults and professionals giving their interpretation of what the child saw and heard. Mixed messages, however, can lead to vision or hearing problems later in life, a way of closing out the untruths and actions they would rather not see. The removal of tonsils in past generations was like a right of passage for many children, but it also forced them to swallow the adult world whether they liked it or not, the throat being the place where reality is swallowed and words allowed to be spoken.

As late as the mid 1980's, surgery performed on babies was done without anesthesia. The doctor's thinking at the time was that the nervous system of babies was not up and running enough to feel pain and that the anesthesia may be detrimental to their health. How unfortunate for them, especially if they lived to carry that imprint of pain throughout their lives. How many children have been emotionally crippled by such things? Children who are now adults. Adults who are now sick. Adults who have no understanding of the relationship of that pain to their present circumstances.

Other patients—20,000 to 40,000 per year in the USA alone—tell of being able to hear and feel everything that happened to them during surgery but that due to the anesthesia they could neither move nor scream. For years the medical profession dismissed such statements as outrageous until it was eventually proven to be true as patients repeated word for word what was said during the surgery. What emotional imprint does the body contain from that pain, that inability to scream, to be heard, to move, being left to endure slow torture?

Children who are given too much responsibility too early in their lives or who endure a traumatic event, often become emotionally overwhelmed in later years which can lead to muddled thinking. Many are labeling with Attention Deficit Disorder (ADD), when it may really be frustration at not being able to grasp what they know is swirling around in their heads. Those who are abused when young often move into a denial mode as a way to close out the pain, sometimes for years or even decades, but while the mind may appear to block it out, the body does not and only when the body finally breaks down, usually as an adult, are the layers peeled back to reveal the true cause of the illness.

We get sick in different parts of the body because our thoughts—energy—congeal in different areas. Everything that has ever happened in our lives, from before birth onwards, is encapsulated in every cell of our being as they record what we see, hear, say and do. And once weakness enters at the cellular level, then emotional involvement follows. This is the critical point where action needs to be taken in order to stop the breakdown before it becomes a full-blown illness.

Aches and pains that we can't exactly pinpoint or even locate within the body, represent a weariness of the soul and a sadness for what life could have been but never was. Once the emotional pain is resolved, the physical problems will lessen too. Even in death the emotions are the last thing to let go, the finally giving up. The organs may have already died, but the mind has to give the body the final okay to leave.

The Muscular System

The bones may be our structure, but the muscles are life itself, and as a system of pulleys and weights the human muscular system is unsurpassed. Comprising approximately 640 muscles, attached by tendons to the bone structure, they do everything from keeping the body alive with air, food and liquids, to holding it in an upright position.

Until recently we understood that the skeletal system, comprising around 300 bones at birth but fusing down to 206 in the adult, was set, and that how strong the overlay of muscles, ligaments and fascia was, was just a matter of good genes, good luck or a good workout. Now, however, we are beginning to understand that what our bodies mature into is what out thought process was earlier, putting a completely new face on body shapes, abnormalities and deformities.

Range of movement comes from flexibility, and flexibility is connected to thought. Do we feel centered and grounded? Are we feeling stressed in our jobs or home life? Do we feel economically secure? Are we unsure which direction to take in our lives? All these feelings are reflected in how our body present itself to the world, and unfortunately in this day and age, very few people have a straight, relaxed posture, an easy gait and suppleness. And rarely do we see kids skip down the street or play jump rope as they once did. Instead, our bodies have become rigid suits of armor protecting us from an unfriendly, hostile outer world—just as countries are also building up weaponry to protect themselves.

Foods and liquids also play their part in the workings of the muscles, and the wrong foods ingested can create a chemical imbalance, which for many people translates into obesity, depression, muddled thinking or other more serious diseases. And in our culture of fast foods and fast living, what our bodies have become is what we have allowed the planet to also become: a toxic wasteland. So, in order to change the state of our health we must first change our relationship to how we grow food to nourish our minds and bodies, along with how we intend to replenish natural resources.

The spinal cord, heart and brain starts to form in the early embryonic stage, making the first couple of months of vital importance to the future development of the fetus. At full term the wiring for a fully functioning being is up and running and ready for action, and as the baby grows, so will its dexterity. The right/left side brain ability comes from the crawling movement of the alternate arm/leg action, so if the crawling time of the baby is curtailed, then it slows the brain's ability to integrate both hemispheres, affecting motor and language skills.

Today many parents, either for convenience or from lack of knowledge, put their baby into a walker where the infant propels itself around by the legs while doing little for the coordination of the arm/leg action that a young child needs to fully develop. The child is then moved from one seat to another as parents strap them into car seats for hours on end and then into strollers—very often well past toddlerhood—leading to lack of muscle-building at a time when the whole system is forming. It also stops the curiosity of the child at an age when children are by nature inquisitive. Once in the stroller, the child is often in a reclining position, making it difficult for them to sit upright and participate in the world around them, which then provokes many to sleep while being pushed. This in turn leads to lack of brain stimulation and creative thinking, which in all likelihood will continue throughout their lives and eventually move many of them into sedentary lifestyles and away from physical activity.

Lack of crawling time can also affect vision, as part of the visual information collected is transferred via nerves from one eye to the other—and eventually one side of the brain to the other—and children who have unattended eyesight problems can experience difficulties with learning and eye-hand coordination.

Many adults also learn by coordinating the hand/ear/eye movements. How many people need to doodle while listening to lectures or in meetings? And how many of the people giving lectures need to pace while speaking, making their alternate leg movement coincide with their alternate brain hemispheres, which brings into question the entire educational system and how we learn?

Poor physical health can come from an unhappy childhood that manifest into muscular constrictions that limits movement in the body as we age, translating emotionally into putting the brakes on future movement in jobs and relationships. Once the emotions start to close down, so too do the muscles as they begin to armor the body for protection. Neuromuscular diseases, which affect how the nervous system fires up the muscles, involve a lack of control over the muscles and our ability to make them do what we want them to do. They are diseases about power and who has the influence over the situation, which could come from an overbearing parent or just our trying too hard to control our own destiny. And as the muscles affects movement, so thoughts also connect to how we enjoy life and our willingness to participate.

When presented with danger, our natural defense mechanism is to tense the entire muscular system, which in cave-dwelling times probably worked well as we sensed danger from wild animals. Now, however, the wild animals are often our own families or the work environment, and the things we are deflecting are words and actions from others. But research tells us it takes thirty repetitions to make something a habit, so imagine thirty times of holding the same muscle group in the same position to combat a negative situation. As those muscles set into what the mind now accepts as "normal," so the distortion of the body begins. Thoughts then start to mold the body.

We each respond differently to any given situation. For some it can be a tightening of the shoulders, for others a tensing of the stomach or constriction of the lungs. At other times the foreshortening of the muscles may start in childhood or in our teen years, gaining an entry point from some physical problem when the body had to compensate for the time that the impediment lasted, but if the muscles "forget" to go back to their original shape, then irregularities in the body begin. They can sometimes take years to manifest into a distortion, and in other cases they are often unseen externally while internally organs may have sagged or distorted in order to compensate, which then starts the armoring and health problems from the inside rather than the outside. The tightening of muscles may be unseen while the body is in good shape, but produces a distortion once the body becomes tired or stressed.

Most of us grow up with some deformity even though to others it may not show, and from childhood onwards we often favor one side of the body more than the other. One of the best places to look for this is in the face, as few of us have symmetrical faces.

Over the past few years as more research about the body structure has been done we are starting to understand that it can change according to which muscle group we work on. Watching the Olympic events is an anatomy class in itself. Swimmers, cyclists, long distance skaters and weight lifters all have very different shapes, as do baseball players, ballet dancers and football players. How the feet turn, in or out, will significantly alter the width of the hip measurement. Ballet dancers' feet turn outwards and their hips correspondingly are slim, whereas baseball players' feet turn inwards, spreading their pelvic area outwards. Likewise, people who push their pelvis forward—which many do thinking it will make their butts look thinner from the side—are actually tilting their pelvis and widening their thighs, and adding to their stomach size as it pushes outward.

Ballet dancers often practice by turning their feet at right angles to their bodies, which not only is an unnatural pose but also makes it difficult to balance. But it does force the body to find its center of gravity (it is very difficult to slouch in this position), which then turns the body into a slim, elongated machine. Martial artists start from a position with the feet apart and knees slightly bent, giving the body stability and grounding and making it hard for an opponent to push them over. In the military, the troops are taught to stand straight with knees locked, which looks good but does nothing for self-defense!

The Body's Emotional Imprint

Cyclists and long distance runners have fairly uniform body shapes, as each muscle group is worked equally. So the sport we push our children into will often determine their body shape growing up, and how we hold our bodies and the patterns we imprint on them, will ordain what distortion we will later engage. If the muscles can be molded into various shapes through sports, given our underlying genetic skeletal coding, then obviously we can do the same thing for our health through that same system by utilizing physical activity and the hands of body workers.

Deformities of the body are a symptom of muscular and emotional tightening, not preordained shapes, and not until we start to release both can the body go back to any kind of normalcy. Without some form of exercise at an early age we are setting the body up for a lifetime of distortions, both emotional and physical, making it even more imperative to give children time to do some physical activity during the day.

But not all sports are equal, and if the body of a growing child is used/pushed unwisely, then the body will rebel years later in the form of pain from that distortion—as many who wanted to become football players can attest as they pop painkillers to mask the pain from adolescent injuries. We don't teach children to listen to their bodies, although we should, but we do teach them to pop pills to alleviate pain.

A positive note is that some schools are now teaching yoga, which is not only good for the brain and physical conditioning, but is also none competitive letting each child progress at their own speed and ability. It also eliminates the dreaded team sports where some child is always the last to be chosen, which is surely why many adults no longer play sports today.

The muscular system is a complex labyrinth that twists, turns and intertwines from the head down to the toes and so any problems with this system, in any area, will affect other areas that we may not think connect to the original health problem. Knee problems can be caused by weak muscles on the forefront of the upper leg, the hipbone or pelvis thrown out of alignment, wrong placement of the feet when walking, or muscle tension in the shoulders or back area. So before opting for any medical intervention it's important to ascertain where the problem really lies.

Aligning and strengthening the spine is the first step in balancing the body and will ultimately lead to a more balanced lifestyle and better physical health.

Words

Family reunions are a chance to catch up with members of the family that we haven't seen for some time, but as the date nears, the initial excitement usually gives way to apprehension as we remember who will say what, and how and who will respond. By the time the reunion ends, silent vows have been taken to never get caught at one again, and to wonder why we disregarded our gut reaction when it screamed "disaster" as we opened the invitation.

Why does this happen? Because our systems have been encoded with a series of buttons, installed by caretakers in our formative years—usually parents and teachers—who, having installed them, know forevermore exactly how to push them. It's like installing a security system in a home and then tracking it once back in the office. And only by knowing the words, or each series of words that each button represents, can we disengage from them. But deciphering the code, as any good safe cracker knows, takes time plus a good memory.

As we replay past family reunions in our heads, it is the words used at those gatherings that are most remembered; words which, depending on whether they were negative or positive, will force our molecular structure to change accordingly. For if we are our thoughts, so too are we our words, as words verbalize the thoughts and form them into concrete existence.

Words can heal or wound, make us weak or make us strong, and which ones we choose to use will depend largely on how we have processed them throughout our lives. They are also an extension of how we function and can kill, cure, make us sick, make us well, or crush the life force from us at any point. Words have power, far more than we ever imagine, and considering how verbal most of us are on the phone, it's amazing how few real words we actually use. Most divorces, we are advised, happen because of lack of verbal communication. Words can also indicate where illness lies without our having any conscious knowledge of it. And the constant use of certain words can also set up illness in the first place.

Many of us now understand that sentences such as "He's a pain in the neck" indicates that the neck and shoulders are where the tension has gathered from the interaction with a particular person, but may not know that constant use of the words, in any situation, can produce that same tension as the muscles become programmed to respond to the trigger words "pain" and "neck". After that, just hearing the name of the irritating person will cause the tightening until eventually the muscles set into a rigid form, holding the body in a constant fight-or-flight position.

"I just can't win with my........" is a sentence many use. But how important is it to win, and at what point in childhood was it set up that we should win? What part of the body is the need to win punishing? And do we really deserve to be punished? How many people have died from heart complications, having complained for years that some situation or person was "breaking their heart?" Or someone complains that there is something "eating away at them," only to find they have cancer. How many boys and girls were told "they'd never amount to anything," and never did? Tell kids enough times that they are stupid and they will be. When we repeat the same words or phrases over and over, we are cementing the emotional patterns of those words into every fiber of our being.

Many people talk of "hanging in" when asked how they are feeling, but imagine a button hanging by a thread and we can guess what they are really saying. And when that statement is made by someone elderly it translates into "I'm barely making it and I need support." The elderly especially, complain that nothing good ever happens to them, but to answer them with another negative, which most of us do to commiserate, only adds to their pessimism. Turning the words back as a positive requires a shift in vocabulary for most of us, but if we answer that their childhood must have been interesting, growing up in (fill in the blank), then it requires a positive memory recall, activating the entire molecular circuit to a positive position— theirs and ours.

When they complain how hard their lives have been, we should remind them of what they did have: food, family, community. Most elderly complain out of fear, fear of getting old and fear of having little control over their lives. But fear is a negative emotion which produces illness, and illness leads to doctors and medication which then reconfirms that they are getting old, making them even more fearful. But the medication is really used to counteract the fear, not the illness.

Surgery is often required to cut away or fix the emotional patterns that have formed into illness or deformity, illness constructed by words and thoughts that loop around our heads day by day, and often, year by year. And even if we do clear the words for a few moments, those same words come back and regroup due to past habits, so in order to regain control we need to use positive words to supplant the old—before they have time to move back in.

Most of us are wounded children who don't understand the depth of the wounds, many of which have come from years of misinformation from those in power constantly telling us that children don't feel, don't understand and don't process information like adults. How many abusive words do children hear and absorb from years of watching television or from hearing abusive songs over and over again? Or sarcastic put-downs from teachers, parents, siblings, peers? Words have a vibrational energy (they are after all sound), and we should choose them carefully according to the kind of energy we want to bring into our lives, and send out to others.

Silent mind-chatter whirls around our minds minute by minute, beating ourselves up as punishment for words we should have said, words we wish we had never said, of actions we wish we had not done and those we wish we had done. The words we hear ourselves saying can also be the most important ones. They are the words we should pay attention to in order to mine information about the truth of our lives, casting light on our emotions and how we are really feeling.

Words can also predict an outcome to a situation beforehand, giving us time to change our actions before they become destructive. "I know I'll fail the exam." "I know I'll get fired for being late again." "I should have taken the other route to work." Walking down the street, sitting at the computer, cooking, taking a shower; we use words everywhere, and once the right words are heard and acted upon, the healing can begin. Words said by others can give us a better insight into what is really happening in their lives too, allowing us a chance to offer the type of support most needed. Kids,

The Body's Emotional Imprint

especially, often don't have words to describe how they feel, which pushes many of them to act out in destructive ways. The frustration they feel inside, then becomes the frustration they feel at having little power in the outer world. How much of Autism is the scream inside that becomes a scream outside as they know that all is not well but have no way to explain it or even how to give the feeling words. This is surely what happens to teenagers as the chaos of the body and mind cries out for release, but they lack a way to release the chaos in a coherent form.

If we say the same words over and over again, then we should heed what body part we are referring to, or what situation or relationship needs attention. Words may also foretell an impending health problem. Hurt emotions can manifest as anger and aggression, but instead of admitting the hurt, we turn it into anger towards others—usually the weaker ones who had little to do with the original upset. Hostile acts come from feeling inadequate, which can also translate into words that are hurtful, so to really understand the emotion that has caused a problem, it is important to see what the opposite emotion would be. Usually anger, hostility and aggression are a cover for more vulnerable feelings such as feeling slighted, humiliated, wounded, useless or unimportant.

Food

So much has been written about foods over the past couple of decades that most of us already know what we should be eating and why. What we don't understand is why we often buy the wrong foods even though we have supermarkets filled with every type of food available.

The great sages throughout time have always known that what we take into our body, through foods and liquids, affects our emotional and physical health. They followed the seasons and ate only what nature provided in that particular season and from that particular part of the world. In the West today we import foods from around the world to eat any time of the year without giving it a second thought. But maybe we should. Our bodies instinctively know that summer time is for light eating, and winter time to add on the bulk, but often, illness is initiated by bucking those rules, either by eating too lightly, or as is usually the case, by eating too heavily for too much of the year.

Today most of us eat on the run, grabbing something from the deli as we rush to work, school and other appointments, something that the body neither needs nor wants. We forego breakfast, making the excuse that we don't have time or don't feel like eating that early in the morning, but then buy something that goes against our better judgment; something sweet, doughy, fattening and convenient but rarely nutritious. By midmorning we usually need to repeat the process.

Physical work that burns calories would make up for the sugary foods, but most of us go to desk jobs where we do little physical activity and that adds to the lethargic, bloated feeling from the sugar fix. Add in coffee and colas, which are acidic in nature, and the brain power for the morning is pretty much shot—to say nothing of setting ourselves up to become overweight and with brittle bones from over-acidity.

It takes 3500 calories to make one pound of fat, so eating 3500 calories less per week would also drop one pound of weight each week—omitting one sugary snack per day over two weeks would give the same results. A large bagel, which most bagels now are, is around 350 calories. One ounce of regular cream cheese is another hundred calories—most people probably have two ounces on a bagel—so together that's 550 calories. Sounds okay for breakfast, which it is, unless you add in a coffee latte at another 180 calories. Then it bumps the number up to around 730 calories, and that's before the day begins. But it's the extra snacks between meals that really add on the calories—especially those late night snacks—the chips, cookies, pretzels, candy bars and sweetened drinks that we consume while surfing TV channels and the Internet.

Our caloric needs are calculated by something called the Basal Metabolic Rate (BMR). This equals the energy expended by our bodies at rest to sustain life—heart beat, organ activity, temperature regulation—all things we never have to think about. These use up to 75% of our daily caloric usage. Another 10% of our daily caloric intake is used to process foods that we consume, which means that if we consume 2000 calories per day, approximately 200 calories goes towards the process of digestion. But our basic caloric needs vary according to our build, height, age and gender, and anything beyond those needs either ends up as weight gain or is burned off by activity. If we balance the calories we use with the calories we consume, then we don't gain weight.

Between 15-40% of our caloric intake is used up on physical activity, so if we walk to work fairly briskly for one hour, we burn off 300 calories. Walk up a couple of flights of stairs and we burn even more, plus we also get a firmer butt. Pushing a lawn mower for an hour burns 420 calories. So save on pollution and health costs and buy a push mower. Then sit back and relax with herbal tea and a couple of cookies—120 calories.

Nowadays, many foods are sold as "natural," but most foods grown are natural! The difference is that many foods have sugars added to them in one form or another, and may also have also been genetically altered (called GMO), which means that they are no longer natural, even though the corporations selling them would have us believe they are. ("Natural" is formed by nature and is not artificial). We are also supposed to believe that the term "natural" is the same as "organic" which again, it is not. ("Organic" is food grown or raised without the use of additives, coloring or synthetic chemicals). Diet foods often have the same amount of calories in them as ordinary foods, but with additives, so get into the habit of reading labels when buying foods and find out what "diet" really means. If it has the same amount of calories as regular foods, then the regular one may actually be more healthful.

A century ago Americans consumed about 6 lb of sugar per year. Now the number has shot up to 100 lb per year—most

The Body's Emotional Imprint

of it from genetically modified corn that has been added, without our knowledge, to all kinds of foods, including packaged French fries, bread, ketchup and a host of other foods consumed daily.

One 12 oz soft drink has the equivalent of 7 teaspoons of sugar in it, although today that sweetener is most likely to be high-fructose corn syrup—again, genetically modified corn. Unfortunately, junk food is often less expensive and more filling than foods with greater nutritional value, and even when salads are available, many of us don't eat them. The only way to counteract the junk food, or even lessen consumption, is to read labels and understand what we are consuming and in what quantities. Eating too much of anything pushes the body out of balance—along with the emotions—and leaves us with continual cravings that the body then has to accommodate.

Buy organic whenever possible and drop the GMO foods altogether. This practice is much more healthful for us and the planet, and the extra cost for organic will more than offset future medical costs. Start to make better choices and the body will respond in kind.

Tune into the body's message—yes, it is sending them. Remember that soda bought from the deli yesterday when the body was screaming "fruit juice"? Most of the time we make our choices by habit, not intellect. We also eat according to the clock, not when the body requires food, which is partly due to our 9-5 jobs.

Constantly gravitating to the same foods, even though we may want something different, requires a weaning process rather than a cold turkey approach. It's much easier to buy the afternoon cup of coffee and cookie if we also buy something healthier too—juice, herbal tea, fruit, protein bar. Think of the coffee and snack as a security blanket until we have the courage to give them up for something more nutritious. Drink less and less of the coffee each week, and buy smaller and smaller cookies. With time, the body won't miss them. And it's a lot quicker to burn a few calories than it is to repair body parts, organs or mental ability.

Everything that we eat and drink passes into the digestive system, and chewing food well before swallowing has many benefits, especially as larger pieces of food take longer to process once in the system. Chewing also increases saliva, which contains enzymes that contribute to the digestive process and aids in the transportation of nutrients once in the body. Plus, eating slower tells the brain when we feel full, which stops overeating and helps in weight loss. We don't tell kids to eat slower, but we should. Or, we do tell them but then lead by bad example by eating fast ourselves.

Herbs are also foods, which we tend not to consider when we take them as supplements, but herbs start off as plants grown in soil and are nourished by water and sunshine. They also contain vitamins and minerals that are beneficial, which is why they are used in cooking throughout the world. Often, people who are not familiar with supplements will complain that when they have taken them, there was no effect. This could be due to the fact that some herbs have fillers, which means they are not pure and fillers are used to cut costs, usually cheaper brands. It could also be because the body doesn't need what is being offered; meaning that it can't utilize the added supplements—like filling a glass that is overflowing. Adding more liquid to to the glass won't help the overflow!

The Body's Emotional Imprint

The wrong foods can weaken the system but the right ones can give us strength to fight infections, bad situations and wrong decisions. And paying attention to health issues will give us an indication of where we are not being nourished, emotionally or with foods, so that we can correct the situation.

Toxins and pesticides can remain in the body for years and have a cumulative effect. The body is a carefully calibrated machine and and in order to keep it at that level and running at high performance, the right nutrients have to be added. If we wouldn't put cheap gas into a good car, why do less for the body?

Right side – Left side

The left side of the body, crossing from the right-brain hemisphere, is considered to contain the more female traits such as intuition, nurturing and creativity, while the left brain, crossing to the right side of the anatomy, represents male traits such as logic, critical thinking and language. The right side is also our public side, the one we are willing to share with the outside world, the left is our private side, the one that is more difficult for people to know.

How strongly we identify with each side often determines how our bodies will form or deform, so it's important to identify which side is pushing, which side is pulling, and which side is winning. Feeling more vulnerable on one side and stronger on the other can cause an imbalance in the muscular system. One leg or arm may become shorter than the other due to muscular stress, one eye or ear may have problems, or subconsciously, we allow one side to drown out the other verbally.

In our culture the right hand is usually the dominant one, forcing us in the past to make left-handed children cross over and become right-handed—and in the process forcing them to rewire their entire system, which labeled many of them slow learners. The dictionary defines left-handed as being clumsy, awkward and insincere, while the right-handed person is considered responsible and to be relied on, so before we even arrive on the planet we have been defined!

We tend to disregard which side of the body, or head, we are having trouble with, and yet each side represents a certain part of our male/female mix. We all have the mix regardless of gender, but in society we have been brainwashed into believing that women who show a more male side are less feminine, and men who have softer female traits must be less masculine.

In truth, we should all be in the middle so that we can connect one hemisphere to the other as desired and needed, but our educational system has almost always been left-brain oriented, even though in the past, school teachers were almost always female. By neglecting right brain traits we have forced those who work better from the right brain—especially women and creative people—to think of themselves as lesser beings in society. Experiments show, however, that children are highly creative before entering school but once they enter the predominantly left-brain educational system, only 10% of the children will be highly creative by age seven, and by the time they reach adulthood the number slips to only 2%. How much of this has contributed to our ill health and the ill health of the planet? If we allowed both the right and left brain to work in tandem, how much better could our society be?

Most of us tend to favor one side more then the other. The pressure of one foot hitting the ground may be more forceful than the other foot. One knee weaker, one hip higher, one arm stronger. Our eyes may vary in size, one ear lower than the other, one side of the face a little different in shape. We may have more trouble with our teeth on one side, the nose may not be straight, the hairline odd. And just as the palm on each hand is different, usually the left being the one we're born with and the right palm formed from our life choices— so each iris of the eye is different, as is each sole of the foot.

When we feel conflicted about some major event or situation, the conflict will often play out by favoring one side of the body more than the other, or will be revealed on one side of the face as the emotions give it form. The way the right and left hemispheres view life and the way they learn and relate to problem solving, will alter the type of jobs that we gravitate to and the relationships we enter into. Problems that develop with our health will also change our physiology, which will change our emotional response too.

When one side of the body breaks down, as after a stroke or paralysis, then we need to also take into account how that side views the world and how we view ourselves in it. Do we feel in control or do we step back and allow others to dominate? Have we taken on our mother's traits or our father's? Have we been influenced by the men of the family, or the women? This goes for both genders.

Men are taught from an early age that real men don't cry, forcing them to hide their more caring side, while women who appear to be uncaring in order to work in a man's world are deemed to have become more like a man. All these things play out in the body and in our health and illnesses as we close down certain areas and strengthen others.

If we choose careers that go against who we really are then eventually our health will suffer. Headaches will arise more frequently, the wrong foods will be consumed, we may gravitate to drugs and alcohol, and relationships will suffer—at home or work.

Paying attention to our left and right side can give us a great deal of information and insight into what area need to be strengthen.

Cancer

The body is made up of trillions of living cells that are the building blocks of life—we begin life as a single cell—and as these cells grow and divide in a controlled way, they produce new cells to replace the old and damaged ones as they die off. Cancer forms when the cells don't die off but continue to grow and divide into new abnormal cells, and having nowhere to go, these unwanted cells form a mass of tissue called a tumor, which can be benign (non cancerous) or malignant (cancerous). Not all cancer cells form tumors, however, as some take advantage of the blood and lymphatic systems to cause their destruction.

Cancer is a group of many related diseases and can form in almost any area of the body. In a healthy individual the immune system can repel invaders, but if the body doesn't have the strength, or will, to fight back, then the place of weakness will allow the disease to take over and increase in size. A traumatic event or someone who is deemed stronger in size, opinion or economic status—family or otherwise—can often start the weakening process, as can a sense of being taken advantage of, or of having little perceived value.

Cancer is a disease of self-worth, as we attack ourselves by growing sickness that devours the good things inside and allows external forces to invade our space. It is the bully

The Body's Emotional Imprint

who expands in the body by pushing aside healthy cells that are needed for life, in order for the unhealthy to grow freely. Cancer cells take up space like invaders, which they are, but invaders appear when the door is left open or when the immune/security system is malfunctioning. Getting rid of them requires the body to build up enough strength to fight back, push them out and close the door.

We weaken ourselves when we place our priorities in the wrong order: too much time spent at work and too little time with family. Or too much family involvement and their demands while our own needs go unheeded. Not enough time spent on the things we want to do while too much time is spend on daily chores which suffocate us. Feeling the need to take on too much responsibility, even though others would probably shoulder some of the burden if asked. Cancer is about imbalance and the inability to know where the balance lies. We often blame external chemicals as the cause of the disease and yet cancer seems to strike indiscriminately: different areas of the world, different family members, different parts of the body.

Being at war with ourselves or with the position we find ourselves in, or the relationship we are in, or just an inability to deal with the life we have chosen, can produce the disease. Also, we may feel the need to be perfect and in control, while the cancer shows who really is in control as it becomes stronger than our own will. It represents our inability to let go of old emotional pattern in order to embrace new and more positive ones. We sometimes retain old patterns to cause pain to others—whom we secretly blame for our unhappiness and lack of confidence—by wanting to make them feel guilty for our disease, and to feel the responsibility that we feel as we become overwhelmed by life. We want them to be better, stronger and more in control in order to counteract our growing weakness.

Unlike many other illnesses, cancer often gives little indication that it is forming until it's too late, and just as we keep our feelings to ourselves instead of voicing our concerns, wants and needs, so a scream builds internally waiting to be heard. It's interesting that cancer is so prevalent today, at a time when we are all fighting for space in an overcrowded world, fighting to be heard when those in power have chosen not to hear. Feeling insecure and fearful as we try to hang onto our own power at a time when Western power is dwindling.

We feel frustration at being held back, especially when we are trying to move to something better but are blocked by others more powerful. We fear an energy crisis as our own energy is in crisis, and experience a spiraling out of control as we reproduce ourselves out of control—just as cancer cells keep reproducing themselves. And just as governments worldwide continue to war, so the war on cancer keeps going too. We are fearful of the future just as much as we are fearful of the doctor's pronouncement that we have cancer. How we interpret the word "cancer," though, can often be the only difference between recovery and falling deeper into sickness, as the cancer changes our intent as well as our molecular structure.

Many believe that cancer is linked to an over-acidic body, while others connect the disease to elevated sugar levels in the blood. An over-acidic body reflects our pH blood level out of balance, which then erodes the bones and affects other body systems. Acid eats into metal and corrodes it, just as an over-acidic body will weaken its own structure. Soft drinks, caffeine, alcohol, grains, dairy, meat, oils, sugar, corn syrup and many pharmaceutical drugs, are acidic—all things we eat and drink in copious amounts. Many of these foods also have a high sugar content. Sugar links to self-love and acceptance of ourselves and others who want to give us love. When we bottle up emotions we dam up the immune system—the lymphatic system—which is the very thing we need to fight the disease with.

Healing crisis

A healing crisis is the turning point of ill health, either emotional or physical, and occurs when the body is ready to eliminate toxins that have remained in the body from some past event or from an overload of toxins that have been stored in the system for a while. As the detoxification intensifies, so a healing crisis often occurs. It can also happen when there is an emotional release connected to a physical action, such as body work, or it can be triggered by taking natural remedies such as herbs, flower or homeopathic remedies, or by fasting or changing the diet to a more healthful one.

Reactions will often mirror the original symptoms that were stored in the body from the time of the event, so if a child didn't have the chance to grieve for a passing parent, then watery eyes, a streaming cold or flu-like symptoms may occur. Other times the healing from trauma can come in the form of a severe headache, nausea, a rash, aches and/or strong emotions such as despair, sadness, fear and anger.

Symptoms can last from a few hours to days, or even weeks, depending on how the child/adult dealt with the original event at the time. They can also vary from very mild to a full-blown illness and can include diarrhea, lack of appetite, a need to sleep, digestive imbalance, visual problems, coughing, skin eruptions, not wanting coffee, alcohol or anything else that would put a strain on the body, and in extreme cases, can cause mercury fillings to fall out of the teeth. Toxins can also be released as a skin rash on one particular part of the body—chest, back, arms, legs—or over the entire body, depending on where the toxins entered and where they rested.

To the uninitiated, when the body does react in some way, the tendency is to stop immediately anything that may have caused the symptoms, but this only stops the detoxification process, so it's important to understand if it is a healing crisis or something that needs medical attention. If unsure, then seek the advice of a professional, but if it is the body healing itself then try and stick with it. Eat light foods, drink fruit juices, herbal teas and broth, and trust the body to instinctively release toxins at its own rate.

A healing crisis may occur more than once, becoming less severe each time until eventually all the toxins are completely released. There is no limit to how much time should pass before a healing crisis occurs. It may be soon after a traumatic event, such as surgery or the ingestion of chemicals, or it may be decades later. It also depends on the person's willingness to initiate one, such as by changing eating habits and being prepared to take some action to detoxify the body in the first place.

The rewards are many—think spring cleaning a home—and include feeling lighter, having more energy, and clearer thinking, with better health and nutrition and a more balanced lifestyle.

Choosing an Alternative Practitioner

C hoosing an alternative health practitioner can be intimidating, which is why most people start by using recom-
mendations. It's a good way to begin, but choosing someone
to help in the quest for better health is subjective, and what
works for one person may not work for another.

A few basic rules to remember:

- A body-worker should be someone you trust, someone
  you feel confident with and someone who is connected
  emotionally.

- Some body workers are excellent technically but lack the
  warmth to convey intimacy—and dealing with a naked or
  semi-naked body is intimate.

- Sexual is not the same as intimate, so know the difference,
  and if it feels sexual, run.

- If a massage leaves you feeling as if you've been hit by a
  truck, the masseuse is wrong for you. It may be the ambi-
  ance, location or vibrations. If the body-worker is unable
  to leave their own emotions at the door, they won't be
  able to accommodate yours—and you're the one paying
  for their services.

The Body's Emotional Imprint

- A good massage should leave you feeling warm, rested and internally glowing. It may also leave you feeling a little drowsy.

- Don't be afraid to walk away and don't be discouraged if the first person you try isn't the right one; it may take five tries.

- Don't think that it's your fault. The reason you are moving towards alternative health care is to take charge of your health and get away from negative emotions.

- Sometimes the connection to the practitioner is something intangible, and yet you will know if it is a little off balance.

- The more you use alternative health care, the more you will tune in to what your needs are, which will then translate into trusting your own instincts. If the practitioner isn't willing to go along with what you think your needs are, and isn't willing to discuss alternatives or a compromise, then find someone who is. It's like going to a hairdresser: if you ask for an inch to be taken off and they lop off four inches because they thought you needed a new image, leave instantly!

- As the work continues, you may feel the need to try someone new. If this happens, it's your body, or mind, telling you to move on. It is nothing personal against the practitioner, but you need change, and change is usually for the good.

- The whole point of using natural health therapies is to give you information that will guide you into the driver's seat. If you feel the practitioner is moving you into a dependent position, then move on. This is not psychoanalysis!

- Many cities now have free health magazines with listings

of practitioners who are good and qualified. If the same name appears week after week, month after month, year after year, then they are still in business, and they remain in business because people keep using their services.

- If you have any reservations about the person listed, then talk to others who use alternative health care and see what their reactions are.

- Don't go by the practitioner's fee. Price, like anything else, is subjective, and someone who is wonderful may charge less than others. Price is often based on their overheads, self-worth, and how much they feel their clients can afford. Many also work on a sliding scale. You want to feel they are on your wavelength, are available emotionally, and care about your health. If they seem reluctant to give out information, especially with regard to your questions, then move on.

- If you are looking for massage or body work, go to someone who is accredited. The wrong type of work can do more harm than good, especially if you have severe physical problems.

- If you are taking pharmaceutical drugs and want to add herbal supplements, or discontinue prescriptive drugs altogether, tell your doctor. He/she should be able to work with you—after all, you want to be in the best of health and they should help you to get there. But be prepared for the doctor trying to discouraged you from going the natural health route, unless they are secure about their own credentials and know something of alternative modalities. You may also have to do your own homework about adverse interactions between pharmaceutical drugs and herbal supplements, which will eventually make you much more knowledgeable about health issues.

The Body's Emotional Imprint

- If the doctor is adamantly against complementary health—and you really do want to incorporate more natural qualities into your health regime, then seek out a medical doctor who is qualified in both mainstream medicine and alternative health. They are out there.

- Many of the larger cities now have natural health expos. Go, talk, listen, get information. Collect anything they give away. Go into health stores and collect free magazines and information; ask questions, read everything you can get your hands on and then begin the quest for more natural health. Whatever you can afford to try, try. The more you know, the wiser the decisions you'll make. It's your body and no one needs to know it better than you.

Health Indicators

The Body's Emotional Imprint

ADRENAL GLANDS

Basic Anatomy

The Adrenal glands, which sit one on top of each kidney, are part of the endocrine system, which by way of the bloodstream are responsible for releasing hormones throughout the body, and for maintaining blood sugar levels. Each adrenal, measuring about 2 inches long and a little over an inch wide, is actually comprised of two glands, one inside the other, with different functions and different fetal origins.

The inner gland, called the adrenal medulla, is responsible for the "fight or flight" hormone epinephrine (also called adrenaline) and norepinephrine, which regulates the heart beat, blood pressure and stress levels.

The outer one, the adrenal cortex, produces hormones that help to regulate the metabolism of carbohydrates, fats and proteins. This gland is also responsible for producing cortisol, which together with corticosterone helps to suppress inflammation in the body, and also secretes dehydroepiandrosterone (DHEA) which is a steroid hormone that converts into testosterone and estrogen once in the body tissue— of particular importance for women as the adrenals are the only source of testosterone. After menopause the adrenals are the only source of estrogen and progesterone, a necessary factor in preventing bone loss, although, before menopause estrogen is also produced in the ovaries.

Emotional disharmony

Stress accounts for a large percentage of all major illnesses, including infections, heart and back problems, insomnia, depression, fatigue, muscle tension, problems in the digestive system and a rise in cholesterol levels. Long term stress also compromises the immune system which can cause other areas of the body to weaken too.

In a perfect world the adrenals would kick in for the time that danger, or perceived danger, is present and then go back to normal afterwards, but in today's stressful world they often never have a chance to go back to the off position. But danger for one person may be adventure for another, so when the body registers fear of any kind, emotional or physical, the stress levels rise and the adrenaline kicks in. A short burst of adrenaline, however, can be beneficial and even exhilarating—think white water rafting—but problems arise when the perceived danger continues.

If adrenals are weakened by stress, they can cause a hormonal imbalance and lead to psychological problems, infertility, and edema or weight loss, but as they also connect to the nervous system, so exhaustion and muscle weakness can also occur, producing an inability to run—physically or emotionally—from a perceived danger. Problems may also stem from past trauma stored in the body that has caused a constant state of exhaustion, especially if connected to a violent situation, or fear that a parent is going to die from illness.

Living with someone who has mood swings and having to constantly be on guard about the right words to use and the right actions to take in order to counteract their moods, can leave the body in a constant state of expectancy and high alert, forcing the adrenals to work overtime. Women are more prone to adrenal problems than men, probably because they are the emotional caretakers of the family, but they are often misdiagnosed as suffering from depression. Adrenal exhaustion for men can sometimes be linked to impotency.

The more stressful our lives have become, the more selfish, we as a society, seem to have also become. But selfishness arises from insecurity and fear of situations we have little control over, and taking care of ourselves first may be the only way we see to take control over the situation. Selfishness is a cloak worn as protection to cover a hurt inside—often from an abusive situation—that manifests as meanness externally. Children often try to protect themselves from bullies by diverting the meanness onto someone who is in an even weaker position, shifting the attention away from themselves. In teenagers selfishness is often related to hormonal changes and is part of the desire to be free from parental restraints and wanting to take more chances—or risks.

When the adrenals are in balance, we feel excited about new prospects and projects, and feel secure in our ability to meet new challenges. We take risks, but the risks are calculated to fulfill our best interest and the interest of those around us.

Words

We talk of being "a nervous wreck" but who, or what situation, has made us nervous? Spouse, parents, coworkers, work-related tension or an overload of things to take care of? Something from the past or the present, or a past traumatic event that has locked the adrenals into overdrive?

Adrenals that are functioning well allow us to cruise through life like a well-oiled car, but once there is an imbalance, they become like a car with the pedal stuck in high gear. We want to make the car stop but can't and at that point we either crash or bail out—neither of which seems a satisfactory option but it will bring attention, and hopefully, some needed help.

Kids who have Attention Deficit Disorder are constantly on the move and have trouble concentrating, but is it really ADD, or just an adrenal or kidney disorder? We tend to think of stress as an adult condition, but children today are put into stressful situations too as they move from one caretaker to another, one uncertain situation to another, one school to another, and often with no one to talk to about their fears. Our lives are now so filled with commitments that we never have time to relax, and that may be filtering down to the next generation.

Listening to the words of children—who are often indirect with their speech—can give us an indication of the real cause of their inability to relax. They may talk about the problems of other kids at school so that the trouble doesn't relate directly to their own fears, but statements such as "Steve's parents are getting divorced and he doesn't know which parent he's going to live with," could be nothing more than small talk—if the parental bond is strong—but it could also illustrate their own fear. "Will my parents get a divorce too, and which parent will I live with?"

President John F. Kennedy suffered from Addison's Disease, a hormonal disorder where the adrenal glands produce too little cortisol. It can cause a bronzing of the skin, which is why many thought Kennedy had an eternal tan.

We usually breathe more shallowly when fearful, reducing the oxygen circulation which can affect the heart and blood pressure. Stress is connected to the heart as it pumps the blood supply around the body. When we are "frozen with fear" the

The Body's Emotional Imprint

words indicate an inability to move away, either from being beaten down, verbally or physically, or from a dangerous situation. But we can also go "white with fear" when we receive a shock and the blood drains from our face. The shock may be from losing money, property or a job, or being left alone to cope with a stressful situation. When we die, the color also drains away, so the inference here is that we are "scared to death."

Young people often say, "I'm charged" or "I'm psyched," pointing to the fact that their adrenaline is pumping and they are ready to go, but on the downside the words can represent an incautious risk taker. Hormone-driven teens will often feel "charged" as they sit behind the wheel of a vehicle, leading them to feel more in control than they really are.

The reverse of this are sentences such as "Oh, I wouldn't dare do that" or "I'm too afraid," indicating timidity and insecurity—words often said by the elderly or by young children who perceive the world around them as too dangerous to participate in. "I'm too afraid to go out," the elderly say as they sense a stressful situation before they even start out, which stops many from being social and enjoying life. And going out in bad weather is especially worrisome, as they wonder, "Will I fall? Will I make it home okay?" before they even leave home. As their stress level increases, so the stress on the muscles also increases as they tense up in anticipation of a fall, which in all likelihood will now happen due to the muscles' being unable to "break the fall."

With kids the words "I don't want to go to school today" usually indicates a problem at school—often with bullies—while the request "let me stay home today, I don't feel well" can also point to a stressful situation with teachers or peers, or with schoolwork that is too advanced.

If the body is healthy, we find ways to deal with physical problems, even if it means exercising to get our bodies in shape for a perceived danger. A weakened nervous system, however, can lead to lack of muscle strength, causing us to feel weak emotionally in dealing with the situation. If we don't "have a leg to stand on," it's difficult to move away from danger. And if we "don't feel up to par" then we don't feel well enough to help ourselves.

Those who are perceived to be weak are usually tormented, and the longer the bullying goes on, the less supported they feel. Children who are small for their age are often at the mercy of bigger and meaner children. The antidote may be participating in some type of martial arts program, which builds confidence as well as stamina. Martial artists, no matter what their stature, learn to use their bodies and minds effectively—rather than using brute force. Participating in some sport or physical activity can benefit all ages and produce a more optimistic outlook as it produces an increase in muscle strength and better heart and lung function.

We speak of someone as "selfish" or doing a "selfish act," but many times that selfish individual has had an insecure and fearful childhood in which they were left to care for themselves at an early age, or had to take care of siblings or other family members. If forced to take on too much responsibility at too young an age, people can develop the desire to hoard, lie or steal in order to take care of themselves first. Often, afraid of not being good enough, they will lie to save face, or allow themselves to be pushed into situation they are unable to say "no" to.

If danger comes from the words of others—threatening words, words that weaken or words that take away physical strength—then learning how to defend against verbal attacks is important. Watching how others navigate through tricky situations is a good way to learn the art of verbal self-defense, as is joining groups where opinions are valued. Learning how to speak up for ourselves and how to ask for what we want is a valuable lesson and one that should be taught to all children from an early age, especially as many of our illnesses are connected to lack of self-confidence.

For many of us, though, the words state exactly what is wrong: "I'm totally stressed out" or "The office was really stressful today." But who was responsible for the situation becoming stressful? Boss, coworkers, family phone calls, an inability to get through all the work? Saying words like this on a daily basis means some action needs to be taken to move away from the situation that is causing the stress, even if it means changing jobs, outlook, or taking the situation in hand by telling the offending party to stop the action that produced the stress—often family members constantly calling, e-mailing or texting. Give them times that they can call, or tell them that they can only make contact at work in an emergency—a real emergency. Constant interruptions wear us down and become stressful as we start to anticipate the calls and texts, which wear away our concentration.

If we are asked to "be brave" when faced with a difficult situation it may entail asking others for help and support. Seeking out others to share the load will reduce the stress level, especially if the load involves caring for an elderly parent and there are other siblings who could help. Facing a severe illness can also put us in the position of having to "put on a brave face" for others when all we really want to do it break down, but breaking down and releasing the emotions will keep us healthier than bottling them up in order to make others feel better.

The repeated saying "I'm exhausted" describe exactly what is meant: mentally, emotionally and physically. The body is "drained" and has no reserve left; in other words, the person is saying, "This is the end and I need help." A cry that should be heeded, either by the one saying the words or the one hearing them, as it implies that they are "at the end of their rope"—which is a dangerous situation to be in.

Feeling "sick and tired" is how we feel after constantly holding our own with someone who won't "give us a break." It's like "going a few rounds" with a boxer. At a certain point the emotions can't take any more punches and the body breaks down and forces a "time out." Compromised adrenals can turn us into a nervous wreck, and then we become nonproductive in all ways.

See Kidneys, Heart, Pituitary Gland, Bladder for additional information.

ANKLES

Basic Anatomy

The ankle is the connecting point between the lower leg and the foot and provides motion and flexibility that allows for movement of the foot. The lower leg muscles and bones, which start at the knee, meet and merge at the ankle.

The tibia, the largest and strongest of the two lower leg bones, also called the shinbone, supports most of the weight when standing, and the fibula is the smaller bone that lies alongside it. Both bones connect at the ankle to the talus, a bone that fits neatly into a socket formed by the tibia and the fibula to form the ankle joint. The talus also connects to the mid foot and the calcaneus—the heel bone—so injuries here affect motion of the ankle and the foot. The talus lacks a good blood supply making the healing of a broken talus bone a long process.

Connecting the outer calf muscles to the calcaneus is the Achilles tendon, which is the strongest tendon (non-elastic connective tissue that attaches muscle to bone) in the entire body and gives the foot flexibility to enable us to rise onto our toes and walk, run and jump. Securing the entire section are bandage-like ligaments, made up primarily of collagen, which wrap around the lower bones and ankle area to give them strength and stability. Problems with walking or running can also come from the hip or pelvic region or from the destabilization of the knees—very often the area where joggers have injuries—both of which can throw off the placement of the feet and weaken the ankle.

Emotional disharmony

The ankle, a bridge point like the neck and wrist, is also the emotional bridge between the legs—forward movement, and the feet—being grounded—so the emotional element is adaptability and having the capacity to give flexibility to both sides. If that flexibility should fail, however, then a fall, sprained muscle or a broken bone may be the end result as one side gives way and the other stands its ground—or at least stands a little stronger than the other side.

A conflict of interest will often present itself if the legs make the decision to move but the feet, which are not sure of the direction to take, remain still. Sprains, which are less serious than broken bones, are usually a subconscious decision to take time out to think about what decision needs to be made, usually something life changing, such as a career move. Or the decision will take care of itself if the injury disrupts a trip or a family or work event .

The ankle stabilizes the placement of the foot, and when in motion is the area where most of the stress is placed. Twisted ankles represent twisted energy—twisting thoughts into knots. When we are in a relationship or a job that is unfulfilling or are conflicted about leaving or staying, we often have weakness here as uncertainty regarding our conviction produces a wavering in our intent. A weakened ankle may then push the foot to turn sideways and cause the body to fall as the dominant emotion that caused the fall prevails. But which side did the twisting and which side received the damage, the right or the left side?

A war between the two sides takes place in most of us until one side wins, and in this area the war may cause one side to buckle under, maybe to another's will. When we make a decision against our better judgment we often ruminate on the choice and don't pay attention to where we are going, causing a mishap. We see the inattention as the problem when it really relates to who makes the decision. There may be a dominant partner in a relationship—marriage, business or friendship—who always gets their way, or someone at work who belittles us and twists our words, provoking us to become indecisive, or we may make a decision and try to change direction at the last minute—walking or driving a vehicle.

Many accidents occur from running down a staircase too quickly, causing the foot to slip and twist. But where is the running to? Somewhere unpleasant? A job interview where we feel unsure of our capabilities? To meet someone we really don't want to meet? Or, are we feeling tired of a situation that is never resolved?

If there is conflict with a job, relationship or marriage, it may force us to take charge of a situation that we don't want to deal with or don't have the means to take care of. In a work environment we could be asked to step back while someone who doesn't have the credentials steps forward, producing conflict in us as we ask ourselves what response we should give: speak up, remain silent, or leave altogether? Sports activities often cause broken or sprained ankles, but is the running the problem, or having to play the sport in the first place? Are we being forced to play when we feel inadequate in that particular sport? Or is the pressure to perform too great?

Ankles, like the knees, holds us in an upright position ready to face the world, but if they collapse, then so too does our world, symbolizing a crisis in faith about certain beliefs. We hit our shin bone—a painful place to hit—usually in the course of moving around from one place to the other, either in an enclosed space that is too small or one that seems too large, reminding us of something or some direction we don't wish to take or move into. Perhaps the circumstances are wrong for us, or maybe the place we are already in is the wrong place, or we are in the wrong job in that space.

Hitting any part of ourselves is a reminder of some negative emotion; anger, guilt, humiliation, not standing up for our rights. But if the problem is caused by a constant weakness on one particular side, then there is a weakness on how we are relating to the masculine and feminine side of us. Perhaps a problem has arisen with our parents and is now playing out as weakened muscles as we try to stand up for ourselves as the parents make us feel weak and vulnerable, just as we felt as a child. Knocking into furniture can also happen to an aging parent as the balance of power changes from the parent being in charge, to their children.

Words

"I don't know whether I'm coming or going" is a perfect example of indecision as we become burdened by too much to do, in too many areas or in too many directions, such as driving the kids to sports, music lessons, and school events. Or, we ask others, "Which way should I go?" or "What do you think I should do?" as we question if it is the right thing to do or not, suggesting the inability to know the right answer. Having the option of staying, going or running, and not knowing which one to choose as the overload in life becomes the overload of the brain at one end and the feet at the other.

Young people sprain their ankles when they are conflicted about their place in society. Considered children on the one hand, but also moving into adulthood on the other, they hover between the two ages—and the two emotional levels. People in a conflicted relationship or with an impending marriage, often have sprained or broken ankles as the clash of emotions merge. They want to run from the situation but also feeling guilty about the action, so the accident gives a time out, a time to think more about the impending event. We usually dismiss the accident as "bad luck" rather than a message from our subconscious to "think before we leap."

We "drag our feet" when we are unable to make an either/or decision to commit an action, finish a project, face a relationship problem, or make a determination that involves others, such as putting an elderly parent into a home

> "Cankles" is a slang word that blends ankle and calf together to describe legs that have no definition from the calf down to the ankle.

versus hiring in-home help. Or whether to take a job with better pay in a different city, or stay in a less satisfying job that gives security.

Playing sports produces sprains and broken bones, especially sports such as skiing, where we lament "I couldn't turn quickly enough," when the ankle really didn't turn in time from the inability to anticipate the turn. As we try to coordinate the feet with the thought process, "should we turn, where should we turn, should we go straight down the hill, do we have the ability to ski to the end?" the conflicted mind then becomes the injured ankle. But what is happening in life that required a turn that couldn't be taken? Or one that should have been taken and wasn't. The ankle break indicates that we should have broken away from the bad situation we were in—violent relationship, abusive boss, stressful job—when we had the chance.

All connective areas of the body are about choice and decisions taken in life. If we feel insecure in taking a direction, about spending money, taking trips, or other things that require a choice, the stumbling and falling takes the initiative and makes the decision for us. "I didn't go on the business trip even though it might have been good for my career."
The legs want to move, the foot wants to stand still, and the ankle hesitates, causing a fall which causes the falling away of the trip.

The ankle is also about "stepping out" and "taking a stand" and "feeling strong." The words relate to how we feel about the lightness of our bodies and to how secure we feel in our lifestyle. Anything that is stopping us from "taking the next step" will impede our forward motion, whether in jobs, relationships or following our bliss.

See Legs, Feet, Right/Left side for additional information.

The Body's Emotional Imprint

ARMS

Basic Anatomy

The elbow is a complex joint at the midpoint of the arm that allows it to bend and pivot as it connects the upper bone, the humerus, to the lower two bones, the radius and the ulna. A ball shape at the top of the humerus allows it to fit into the shoulder socket to provide for rotation of the arm, while the radius and ulna bones, which start at the elbow and end at the wrist, are wrapped in ligaments to hold them in place.

The rotor cuff, a group of tendons and muscles in the shoulder that fan out from the humerus to the scapula— large triangular shaped bones that lie one each side on the upper back—give stability and action to the shoulder. Weakened rotor cuff tendons, which attach to the humerus and give the joint durability, can detach due to an accident, repetitive action, age or general wear and tear.

The muscular system of the arm is an intricate web of intersecting muscles that weave their way in, out and around the bones to connect the arm to the shoulder and across to the chest and ribs. Any foreshortening of these muscles can produce a tightening in the arm and a restriction of movement. For a full range of movement, all the interconnecting muscles must be unrestricted—front, back and side.

Strong bones are also needed to provide strength to the arms, as the bone tissue, which lies inside the bones, is the main mineral reservoir for storing calcium and phosphates until needed, and for helping to remove heavy metals and other foreign elements from the blood.

Emotional disharmony

Arms embrace life, loved ones and the world around us. They represent expansive thinking—as we gesture the distance with outstretched arms—or produce limited vision, restricting the length of the arm movement as they withdraw back to the body, tightening the shoulder and chest muscles as they go. An inability to move the arms up and out is usually seen as a problem with the arms themselves, but often it is the shoulder muscles connected to the chest and back muscles that cause the constriction. The arms connect to the shoulders, where movement pivots from the sockets and gives them freedom to move back and forth, swing out to the side, or up into the air and down into the ground.

Depending on our emotional well-being, we use our arms to hug, embrace, give consolation and hold. But we can also hit, shake, lift or push down, depending on how we feel about ourselves, and our life, job and relationships.

The act of embracing is very emotional for many people, especially those who were not brought up in demonstrative families. Children who were pushed away by parents tend to be more guarded in their show of affection than those who were encouraged to use their arms to show love and happiness. But if we feel shy about embracing others, then we will probably be just as shy about reaching for what we want in life. Our bodies reflect our emotions, although, some forms of openness are little more than a gesture of civility, which is common in political and business circles. For most of us, though, arms are used to express emotions of joy and expansiveness.

This area is where the energy of older people is often blocked, which leads to lack of movement and an inability to lift heavy objects or to straighten an arm or put their arms above their head. As they withdraw from life, a gradual closing down to the outside takes place until they are unable to reach out for the things and people they want. Sometimes the withdrawal comes as a reaction to others who, seeing them age, no longer want to embrace them, causing the elderly to close themselves down even more and restrict their movement as they take in the rejection. Children often don't like to embrace older people as they see them being very far away from their own age group and that of their parents, making the elderly feel unwanted by the very people they most want to be accepted by.

Sprained arm muscles come from overreaching as we move towards things we fear are too big for us to handle, at work, in relationships or in love. Broken arm bones reflect a break of energy, a breaking in two, a snapping of the bone as it weakens. But who or what has weakened it? Spouse, boss, parents, unkind words, unkind actions? Is the break on the left or right arm? Does the break or sprain connect to a new relationship or a new job that has made us feel vulnerable, insignificant, or out of our league? Any wound to the arm represent fear of embracing what we love. Do we love our jobs, love our spouse, feel love for the world? Do we feel safe in expressing our affection, or do we feel anger and hostility at having to—a holdover from childhood as we were made to kiss parents or other relatives we didn't want to hug and kiss.

Most of us have a dominant arm, one that is a little more muscular than the other and is usually connected to whether we are predominantly left- or right-handed. If we are in a job where one arm is overused, then it may be throwing the whole body out of balance, affecting the spine down into the pelvis and leg area. Athletes often suffer from an imbalance in their bodies from using one leg or arms more than the other one, as do people who do heavy manual work.

Holding the arms crossed over the chest is a sign of not allowing others to get close as we keep everything inside and protect the heart from hurt. Crossing the arms across the body is also an act of embracing ourselves when we need reassurance, but it also pulls the front of the body inwards while the back becomes rounded like a turtle as we retreat back into our own shell.

In a work environment, arms across the chest can also represent a nonverbal sign of disagreement with someone, usually those with a higher status than ourselves to whom we feel unable to voice our opinion, and in order not to be confrontational we hold the words firmly inside, not allowing them to escape for fear of reprisal.

The forearm muscles, the main muscles between the elbow and the wrist, are most often the ones strained from carrying things that are too heavy as we find ourselves unable to give strength to the action. But is the item really too heavy or is the problem the content of that is being carried? Is it a child that has become too heavy to hold or an inanimate object that is no longer needed? Is the item being moved from one location to another, and is it to a better or worse location? Or, perhaps, there is resentment at having to carry things for others? Or having to move to a different location or office?

Any damage to the arm when doing an action is an indication that we hold some kind of resentment at having to do it, or are fearful of moving into some new situation. Sometimes we push away the very people we most need in our lives, and that too can affect the arms as we bruise, cut, sprain them or break bones from the guilt, anger or unhappiness that we feel. The lower arm represents the holding, while the upper arm moves upwards and outwards—but only as far as we accept both ourselves and others.

If we feel confident and happy about life, however, we let our arms swing each side of the body as we walk. This is an outward sign that all is well and we feel secure about taking up enough space for our needs. The head is erect, the back straight, the walk easy—and the arms are free and swinging as we go forwards.

Words

The arms are very expressive, even without words, but when we add in the words, we show how we feel at certain points in our lives, and how much we welcome the exterior world. Do we want to give freely or withhold? Expressions like "Oh, I could have hugged them!" usually come from someone connected to humanity and who has a willingness to connect person to person, while negative words such as "He needs slapping down" or "putting in his place" indicates a desire to use physical force to deal with an emotional aggravation. Men who only know violence as a way of dealing with problems, usually say things that include blows or beatings like "I'll beat him within an inch of his life," "He deserve to be kept down," or "He deserves to be laid out." Physical violence seen as the only outlet for their anger.

But arms are also for lifting and when we see others doing the "heavy lifting" and feel shame at shirking our responsibilities, it can produce an injury to our own arm later on as the guilty for not participating takes form. "I should have helped them when I had the chance" is the unsaid implication. Injuring our forearm muscles lifting an elderly parent or relative who is ill, can come from resenting the fact that other family members are not doing "their part" or "pulling their weight" on the project, or won't help pay the medical bills.

Those who have little confidence in their abilities talk of ideas and things in terms of size. "The idea/job was just too big," they say with a gesture of spread arms to show that their vision stopped at the same point their arm width stopped. Others, who embellish the truth, also use their arms to show the size of what they have accomplished, or think they accomplished, as their outstretched arm encroach into the space of others.

> Those who are willing to roll up their sleeves and "get stuck in," are usually much more relaxed about situations than those who keep their cuffs firmly "buttoned up." Clothes tell a lot about people.

On the other hand we tend to use elbows aggressively as we "elbow others out" of things or situations that we want for ourselves. But is it really necessary to elbow others out or is there a better way to get what we want? Perhaps "killing them with kindness" would give us a better result—and be better for our image. Elbows are hard and sharp, and "She elbowed me out of the way" reflects the sharpness of the elbow instead of the sharpness of the tongue.

Religions teaches us to raise our open arms towards heaven as a way to give praise to a supreme power, a way of accepting that there is something much higher than ourselves. And when we give thanks, we often give the same gesture, as if we have been given what we asked for.

We may talk with our hands, but the arms show the degree of frustration or accommodation, which is shown by the placement of the elbows—close to the body indicates exasperation while further out shows a more forgiving nature. Older people complain they can no longer "reach" for things, but that usually accompanies other muscular restrictions like the legs and pelvis as the muscles begin to weaken, too.

We talk of illness as something "I just couldn't shake off" as the sickness lingers on. We want to shake it away but are unable to do so due to a weakened body, or a weakened will. But we also say "I just couldn't beat it" when a more aggressive action than shaking is needed to reduce more severe symptoms. We also use the word "shaking" for actions we want to do to others as we say, "I'll give him a good shaking," which translated really means that we want them to do the action in order to satisfy our own needs.

Arm gestures can be kind or unkind, and which we choose will depend on how we feel about our own lives as we move out into the world and connect to others. Some actions are used as signs of defiance such as one arm raised with fist clenched—a form of salute to indicate belonging to a group or cause. But we can also wrap our arms around others as an all encompassing action bathed in compassion, and if given with a smile is universally accepted as a gesture of goodwill. And saying, "I will embrace life" is to let go of all the negative emotions that are holding us back, allowing us to embrace people, situations, a new lifestyle.

See Shoulders, Chest, Wrist and Hand for additional information.

BLADDER

Basic Anatomy

The bladder, a muscular sac about the size and shape of a pear, is located in the pelvis area just above and behind the pelvic bone. In adults it stretches to accommodate around a pint of urine, passed down from the kidneys to remain in the bladder until it is discharged through a tube called the urethra—about 8 inches long in males as it passes through the penis, and 1.5 inches long in women.

The sphincter muscles are circular muscles that form around the opening of the bladder into the urethra; they help keep the urine from leaking and also stimulates nervous impulses to indicate a need to urinate. The bladder muscles then contract, forcing urine to pass through the urethra. The amount of liquid expelled depends on what type of fluids and foods have been consumed and how much fluid has been lost through perspiration, urination and respiration—although too much liquid loss and not enough replenishment can result in dehydration and acidosis—measured by pH numbers that indicate the balance between acidic and alkaline levels.

Normal urine color can go from pale yellow to a deep amber (although eating beets will produce red urine). The color depends on the type of foods eaten, the amount of liquids taken in, and how healthy the individual is. If in good health, urine should produce little to no odor.

Emotional disharmony

The urinary system keeps water and chemicals, such as potassium and sodium, in balance, and allows the liquid to flow at an appropriate time. How the liquid flows, passing easily or with difficulty, indicates how freely our emotions are flowing too. As the liquid also connects to the kidneys, having passed along from them into the bladder for the final release, so the emotions of fear, uncertainty and worry are also shared.

Incontinence and bed-wetting produce worry and apprehension as the urine is released at inopportune times, and if the problem persists, so fear and anxiety will also increase, leading to greater lack of control, and a spiral of mounting fear as the problem begins to restrict movement from the home base. Inability to control the stream of urine, however, is produced by the weakening of the muscles that allow the bladder to open, close and expel the liquid, and so it reflects an inability to control the flow of life and the outcome. It is the final receptacle of our inner worth and how that inner worth relates to the outside social society, and whether we feel worthy of participating in it.

Many children wet their beds when the natural mechanism that usually alerts them to the need to wake up and urinate, fails. So what in their life do they feel they have so little control over? Is life overflowing with too many things going on at once, too many things to take care, or are they growing up so fast that they are unable to grasp the lessons needed to take the responsibility?

Or, for some children, the fear—and bedwetting—may come from the home environment, with fighting parents or divorced parents who often leave the child uncertain of their home base, or the death of a parent or sibling. Fear of being homeless can have the same effect on both the young and the elderly, especially if they are asked to move homes, either to a new area and school and away from friends and relatives, or to a totally new environment, city or country. In older people incontinence is often associated with having to move into an assisted living home away from friends, or the fear that they will eventually have to move as their ability to care for themselves decreases.

Bladder infection known as urinary tract infections (UTI) or cystitis, is an inflammation of the bladder, usually due to infection, which affects most women at least once during their life, although it does affect men too. Due to the shorter length of the urethra, women usually contract it from sexual intercourse as the bacteria in the vaginal area is pushed into the urethra. But what is the inflammation/anger from? What emotion is the bladder releasing that is causing such pain? A marriage that is over and we now fear being alone?

The bladder is also part of the genital area and is connected to the emotions of that space too—often negative feelings related to sexual relations with an unfamiliar partner, or someone we are not comfortable with, or, in many cases, when the message passed from female family members was one of prudery and disgust at the sexual act and the idea that women have no right to enjoy it.

Infection anywhere in the body is an indication of weakness and vulnerability, but in the genital area it indicates a lack of trust, or an unreadiness to have a sexual relationship. A recent marriage will often bring up emotions in this area, which is why many women develop cystitis during or right after their honeymoon.

Words
The bladder, being a sac, is about containment and being in control of our watery emotions. Often, what we really want

to do is to be overemotional and "have a good cry," but instead we try and "hold it all in" so that others are not offended. We try not to spill it in inappropriate places or at inopportune moments, fearful that we will be labeled too emotional about events that are either happening or about to happen. This applies especially to women who try not to be overemotional in a work environment, or try not to go to the bathroom when the need arises.

"Spilling the beans" because we are not able to contain the information passed along or not wanting to accept the words others are saying, or the responsibility of having to keep a secret, can represent too much responsibility that has become a burden. Perhaps too much responsibility was placed on us as a child and we had no way of controlling it.

If the muscles of the bladder are strong then we can let the urine go when we are ready. If not, then it isn't our decision to take—or so we may feel. Someone in authority may be

> A teaspoonful of baking soda in juice or water is a quick way to bring the body back to an alkaline state.

making the decisions for us and we feel duty bound to follow them: doctors, family members or a caretaker. A spouse may take charge and leave us with little choice in the matter, or a sibling may start making decisions with regard to the future home of an elderly parent.

"I had to let it all out" or "I just couldn't hold on any longer" indicates a tiredness about a situation that we feel incapable of fighting—especially if incontinence is a factor and we are too tired to "put on a brave face" any longer, which is why many elderly often let their appearance go too. Their dignity is already compromised, so why bother?

If we are constantly stressed and feel "completely drained," or talk of others who have completely "drained" us, we mean that we are so tired of the situation that we no longer have the energy to care what others think. Draining can sometimes be a good thing if the situation is able to drain away, but liquid that backs up usually cause problems later on. We drain land in order to allow a building to go up, producing something useful, but if the land isn't well drained then the land will flood when the rain arrives. Keeping our urinary track in good working order will allow the unwanted emotions, words and situations to drain away at the appropriate time.

Cystitis makes it painful to pass liquid and gives a feeling of constantly wanting to urinate, even though very little liquid is passed each time. Having little control over the bladder, or feelings that have bottled up, stops the flow and causes a blockage that won't release the liquid, or us, from the circumstances we find ourselves in. But is the fear real or imagined? Is it an obsession about something that will never come to pass? About a humiliating situation, or a fearful one? A situation that happened well before the pain started but was triggered by another, similar and humiliating experience? We tend to "hang on" to humiliating experiences, often for years, even though the people or person associated with the incident have moved on. For us, though, the imprint is something that we can't let go of, and the cystitis is a painful reminder of that.

Kids talk of someone who has "made me pee in my pants," which could be a good experience when they laughed too much, or one where they were fearful. So who was doing the action—usually tickling—to make them wet themselves? Someone they trusted, or someone they disliked? Someone who took delight in humiliated them as they urinated over themselves, or someone who loved to see them laugh and tickled them as a kind gesture? Not all laughter is good laughter. We laugh when we are embarrassed and we laugh when we want to be polite. So check if the person is friend or foe, especially if it concerns children.

Money is associated with the bladder too, as it tends to flow out of our lives at a quicker rate than it flows in. Spending money we don't have will often leave us crying that "I've pissed away all my money" or are "pissed off" by someone who has annoyed us for things we have really done to ourselves. We may have squander money needed to pay bills, but "letting it all go" feels so much better emotionally, if not practically.

Other times, we just "won't let things go" and hang on to people, things and situations out of fear of being alone, then fight against letting them flow along naturally, which causes bacteria to grow into a bladder infection just as the clinging has caused ill will to grow against the people concerned. Force of will and the need to take charge, no matter how detrimental the outcome, has now caused us pain.

"Going against the flow," though, suggests we are strong enough to do whatever we have set our minds to, in this case, being able to stop the flow whenever we need to, suggesting that we are in charge of the decision. The flow of urine is the flow of all that is negative and unwanted as we empty the bladder to allow the fluid to leave at the appropriate time. Sometimes others will not allow a problem to flow out and block our way, forcing us to worry and to "hold it all in," instead of dealing with the situation that is blocking us. Unfortunately, health problems related to the bladder often come before the words are spoken or the matter attended to.

"Treading water" means remaining in one place and can apply to an actual location or job, or to negative emotions that arrive as fast as we move them out. Maybe someone close to us, either at work or at home, won't leave us alone and the anger builds as we are unable to release the words to stop the "flood" of calls and e-mails. People who "drain us" are demanding people who need attention and drain energy, money or resources. The end result, of course, is that the one who has allow the draining to happen is "left holding the bag" with their resources drained, while the one who did the draining continues on. Elderly people who are lonely, will often allow others into their homes for companionship, and are then taken advantage of by those who feel no compunction about deceiving them.

Feeling the need to urinate constantly may result from wanting to purge the situation from our lives, especially if it involves negative people who "drain our energy."

See Kidney, Ovaries/Uterus and Prostate Gland for additional information.

BOWELS – Hemorrhoids

Basic Anatomy

The bowel is part of the elimination process and is the lower portion of the digestive system, also called the gastrointestinal tract. The rectum, a small tube about 6 inches in length, is the final part of the colon and the storage place for feces before elimination takes place. The entire system from mouth to rectum is around 25 feet long.

Fecal matter is pushed through the colon by contracting muscles that move in a wave motion called mass peristaltic movement. This action is controlled by the autonomic nervous system—an automatic action requiring no conscious thought.

From the colon the matter moves into the rectum, where it forms into stools and then passes into the anal canal ready for evacuation from the anus. As the urge to defecate increases, two sphincter muscles, the internal and external, allow the anus to open and dispose of the feces. The internal muscle releases the feces into the short anal canal—about 1 inch long—and the external muscle, a circular shape at the anal opening, allows the expulsion of the fecal matter.

A healthy person should have have 2 to 3 bowel movements a day, shortly after each meal, but in today's world, where people work long hours outside the home, the body is usually trained to eliminate once a day for convenience. Stools should be light brown in color, although the color can vary according to the food eaten, and should be long and dense with a large diameter and no offensive odor. Generally, stools that are too hard means there isn't enough fluid in the system; if they are too soft, there isn't enough roughage in the diet.

Hemorrhoids, also called piles, are inflamed veins around the anus and can be internal or can protrude from the opening walls. Most hemorrhoids shrink back on their own, but those that protrude permanently may require treatment. The cause of the inflammation and swelling is usually from straining during bowel movements, but pressure on the veins during pregnancy and delivery can also be a cause, as can irregular bowel habits such as constipation or diarrhea, exercise, obesity or sitting for long periods at a time.

Emotional disharmony

A bowel movement is letting go of food waste after all the nutrients have been removed and used, the natural progression of waste at the final point of the digestive process. An unnatural release will show itself as either diarrhea or constipation, so how we really feel about releasing all the unwanted emotions and waste in our lives is indicated by how the feces evacuate. Are the stools too loose, too hard or well formed? Do we want to release them too quickly, as in diarrhea, or hang onto them for too long, making us feel uncomfortable as we become constipated? What emotions are we holding on to that we should give up? What is it that we refuse to give up, but is causing us pain? Or, who is causing us pain? What words are we hanging on to that should be released? Who are we holding on to that we should have let go long ago, and why is it so difficult to let them go?

Constipation represents information not being processed in a timely manner, which we hold on to when it should have been passed on and out—maybe to others—a long time ago. Waste that comes streaming out in an unregulated, unformed way as diarrhea, denotes the inability to let a matter form as it rushes through us before we have time to digest the implications.

We get food poisoning from food that is infected with bacteria, causing us to want to release it as fast as possible. It forces us to step back from all that is going on while we "get it all out" of our system. If the immune system is strong, then the food poisoning will be weaker and allow us to get back and participate in life much sooner. But what did we eat, and who were we with when we ate the offending food? Were we alone or with someone who was disagreeable? Where were we when we ate the food, in a restaurant or in someone's home? Who is causing us to suffer as we are unable to digest the implications? What is flowing through our life before we've had time to address it? What are we too afraid to look at and deal with?

As diarrhea is connected to the digestive process, the implication is that the nourishing food is pushed through too quickly to be of any benefit to us. We are, in fact, rushing it through without being able to receive the nutrition/love that others may want to give us—especially those who have provided us with the food. Or, perhaps the food is given in exchange for something else: favors, love, sex, companionship. Diarrhea, often a watery mess, is a poisoning of the system that affects our ability to function. A desire to get rid of the poison—people, situations, family members—as fast as possible, or those who are forcing us to rush through a matter without taking the time to think it through first. It is also about the feces not being fully formed or our not allowing them to form fully for an easy evacuating. So what information do we need to gather in order to form a conclusion that would benefit all parties?

Many older people have trouble evacuating and yet because they have problems with flexibility they put another toilet seat on the existing one, making their posture more one of standing than sitting and making evacuation almost impossible. In many cultures—and with our ancestors too—squatting was and is, a natural way to eliminate until we invented objects to sit on. But as we raise the toilet seat higher and higher, we also raise the difficulty of letting things go, often causing constipation. Not being able to sit is usually caused by lack of flexibility and muscle strength and leads to lack of movement, but what are we being inflexible about that is making it too difficult to perform a natural task? Daily life that is too punishing and tiring? Too much to handle? Was there something that had to be held in for safe keeping but should have been dealt with years ago? Secrets revealed that now can't be passed on and out? Relationships that should have been sorted out but never were? Finances that should be dealt with but never will be?

Constipation is a holding back, a feeling of insecurity which is often related to money and the direction life is taking. It is a need to hold on to things and people just in case there is nothing more coming, producing a distrust of others or of our own ability to cope with the ups and downs. It can be a hoarding mentality that blocks the system, stopping money, or anything good, from coming in to be processed, used, and then allowed to leave again, or a fear that more won't be arriving, which usually results in less coming back. Money, love and possession are all closely linked to how secure we feel about the things we need to survive.

Many who are constipated use a laxative in order to release the feces, but eventually the laxative weakens the colon and does nothing to confront the real emotional cause of the constipation. Some have only one bowel movement every few days, causing the waste matter to turn putrid, which is how the emotions eventually turn as the blockage results in a bad temper, rigid thinking and a refusal to see a different point of view. We feel a sense that life has passed us by, leaving nothing more than negative emotions, which we allow to restrict us, just as the colon also becomes more and more restricted.

For some, bowel problems go right back to toilet training during childhood, which was a way of controlling caretakers. Withholding feces is often the only power the child has, and is usually no match for parents who do have the control. On the other hand, feces can represent something dirty, something not spoken of, making it difficult in later years to allow life to progress naturally. Is there someone holding back on an issue that needs to be resolved, or are we the one holding back the information so that a conclusion is never reached, perhaps to get back at someone—partner, spouse, parent— or to keep someone in our life who will leave if the issue is settled.

Hemorrhoids itch, often with a burning sensation, and usually result from pushing too hard to evacuate. A desire to get rid of something even though the problem, and emotional involvement in an issue, won't leave, like a nagging that won't go away. But nagging things are usually small things—as are hemorrhoids—that we don't want to deal with. So, what is that small irritation that needs attention? Or are we the nagging one, nagging others to do what we want? It is about letting go, but with a lot of aggravation and anger to accompany the final release. So who or what is the itching from? What, or who, needs scratching out of our lives, and why are they so difficult to get rid of? Is there a complication in a relationship, such as a long divorce? Someone who refuses to leave us alone—a family member, in-laws, ex? If the hemorrhoids are outside the anus, then the irritation has moved beyond the surface and could become a major problem requiring surgery and forced intervention by an outsider—leaving them to make the final decision that we seem unable to make.

Irritable bowel syndrome (IBS) is caused by taking on too much responsibility at too young an age and not allowing our true feelings to surface, which forces the feelings to remain inside as the bloating increases. As the bowel habits swing from diarrhea to constipation, so the feelings of responsibility clash with the need to be irresponsible. One side pushing the other, with our true feelings squashed between. It can also come from an irritating situation or person that we know will not leave us alone, perhaps a parent or spouse that we will never be totally free from simply because we do feel responsible for them—and they know that.

Words

In Western culture, swear words refer to bodily functions: *shit, crap, merde,* and other derogatory terms are used to describe how we feel about things, people and situations. Wanting "to get rid of all this shit in my life," states that it is no longer a small aggravation, it is a proclamation of wanting to eliminate everything and everyone who is causing, or adding to, the perceived problem. We feel tired, burdened and need to move on. Aggressive people talk of "beating the crap" out of someone. The victim isn't killed but their bodily functions are damaged so that they will never cause trouble again.

Bullshit is a term we use for others who stretch the truth, as in "he was such a bullshitter" or who" talks a lot of bull."

Bullshitters like to feel in charge, which is how we feel as toddlers as we were being toilet trained. The feces then become either a reward to the one in charge, or a mess that has to be cleaned up by the one in charge. So are we below, and accepting the bullshit, or above the situation and can see through it?

"The guy doesn't know his ass from his elbow" implies someone who is in charge but who isn't doing a good job. We often say it about coworkers or a boss, and it stems from the frustration of not having their position but feeling that we could do a better job if given a chance. But who has the bowel problem? The one we are complaining about or ourselves? If we are the one with the problem, then it is up to us to address that fact and take control, even if it means "speaking our mind," or leaving the job, marriage, partnership—or we continue to have bowel problems from the resentment that keeps building.

The elderly often have constipation problems as they age. They fear releasing what they have—money, autonomy, health—as they try to gain control but confirm that they are "afraid to spend the money," or afraid to "give up my home." At the end of life, the opposite happens as the body—and muscles—can no longer control the bodily fluids and so release them.

Irritable bowel syndrome (IBS), as the name suggests, is an irritation in the lower part of the digestive tract that comes and goes repeatedly. The gut is connected to the brain, so who or what is causing the irritation? Check when each episode occurs.

Bowel problems are about being conflicted. We experience a swing of emotions as the body tries to find middle ground.

We know a problem should be released, but are not able to release the feeling of anger and hurt connected to it. Or, we find ourselves caught in a conflict where we are the one who must find a solution, but become upset as we know that no solution will be acceptable to others. Maybe a boss who is expecting a response, or a group who awaits a reply, or a family member who refuses to see our point of view. In our stressful society the problems affect us by not allowing all the irritations of life to pass through and out.

Sometimes we are "itching to tell the truth" and have a burning desire to say something but know that we can't. Wanting to release the words but not being able to do so, we "sit on them." But what are we protecting and what will happen if the words are released? Is it our truth, or do the words/secrets belong to others? Is it a work- or home-related situation? Releasing the words may be better for us and our health in the long run, but may cause eruptions, or disruptions to others, so is it worth taking actions now, or is there another way to deal with the situation without anyone getting harmed? What words can be said that won't accuse and will not let the situation flare into something that will cause dis-ease to all?

The "fiber of life" represents strength, but the lack of fiber in our diets, can produce hemorrhoids as we strain to release the waste. We also talk of "lack of moral fiber" when we see weakness in others, but it can also be weakness in ourselves at not having enough substance to face a problem. Fibers are long strands that are strong and resistant and suggest a strong resolve, and so having a "strong moral fiber" means we are willing to stand up for our rights. Unfortunately, when we don't, hemorrhoids—and anger—can appear in place of the strong fiber. We keep trying to do the right thing, even though it is getting "harder" to do, and resentment grows when we have to put our "best effort" into things for others and not ourselves. That's when we "push back" and free ourselves.

See Colon, Pancreas, Intestines and Mouth for additional information.

BRAIN -Alzheimer's – Tumors

Basic Anatomy

An adult male brain weighs about 3 pounds, the female brain a little less, and is the central control room for the nervous system—the transmitting and receiving of messages for the workings of the entire body: movement, behavior, senses and intelligence.

The brain is divided into three main areas. The *cerebrum* consists of about two-thirds of the brain's volume and is divided into the left and right hemispheres, joined by a thick bundle of nerve fibers called the corpus callosum. Each hemisphere consists of a core of white matter surrounded by gray matter called the cerebral cortex, and is responsible for personality, thinking, reasoning, emotions, memory, speech and problem solving.

The second part, the *cerebellum*, accounts for 10% of the brain's volume but contains over 50% of its neurons and is responsible for maintaining balance, equilibrium and fluid movement.

And finally, the *brainstem*, which links the brain to the spinal cord and coordinates the messages crossing them over from one side to the other—the right side of the body governed by the left side of the brain and vice-versa—to carry out the appropriate action. The brainstem is responsible for all vital life functions: breathing, heartbeat and blood pressure, and also for sensitivity to pain and consciousness. All information relayed from the body to the brain must pass through the brainstem.

The brain is fed by oxygen and glucose, and although it weighs only 2% of the body's weight, it consumes 20% of the energy produced by the body. Brain cells deprived of oxygen will die in less than four minutes, and if deprived for less time, they can adversely affect all, or part, of the nervous system and the working of the entire body, externally and internally.

Emotional disharmony

The brain is the center for the nervous system and is the messenger network for the entire structure, receiving information and sending it out to the appropriate places for particular actions to take place. For this reason, the brain affects both the psychological and the physical aspects of who we are and how we function.

Accidents can result in wounds and trauma to the brain from an external force hitting us, while tumors build from the inside and are the result of tangled thoughts that have no outlet. As the tumor grows, so it forces the brain to make room for the mass, pushing aside other vital areas.

Problems with the brain can stop people dead in their tracks, just as tumors stop ideas and thoughts from being acted upon. Very often those with tumors have had restraints placed on them by society or others around them—to be responsible people and to muffle imaginative and innovative ways—when all they really wanted to do was toss it all and walk away. Tumors can occur at any age, even in very young children, and just as the cranium, which contains the brain, can only grow to a certain size, so thoughts are also contained within that same space.

Those with tumors and other brain disorders—or even people who think a lot but don't act on their thoughts—are often described as living inside their heads. Unable to verbalize their true feelings or ideas, they retreat to a place where thoughts have a safe haven; safe from unkind words spoken by others who lack understanding, and safe from those who attack their ideas. Often feeling unacknowledged, they retreat into themselves, which allows them to role-play and become who they believe themselves to be—usually misunderstood but brilliant beings with thoughts and ideas they are not allowed to say or implement. They may lack emotional support for their endeavors and be constantly put down for having silly ideas, which forces them to carry all their ideas around until they can bring them into concrete existence.

Alzheimer's disease is about forgetting; the names of those they love, the people they know, the route they take home, the layout of their own homes. It's an abdication of responsibility as they regress back into childhood to be taken care of and told what to wear, where to be, what to eat. Many who succumb to the disease have been the support of the family for most of their lives—and have silently resented the situation they found themselves in. Now, finally, they are the one being taken care of. Very often, they were the emotional support for the family, and often unrecognized. We can see financial support in physical terms but emotional support and the people giving it are often undervalued, the same way women who were homemakers were undervalued.

When things occur in life that are distasteful, hurtful or traumatic, we retreat into denial and close down all memory of the event or events, and Alzheimer's is a slow closing down, a wanting to forget, a giving up and not caring about anything and no longer needing to. Now they have a legitimate excuse not to. For some, there is anger and aggression, pent-up anger finally unleashed on family members and friends. They can lash out and not feel responsible for their harsh words—words they have wanted to say for a very long time.

Brain lesions result from the wearing away of the brain function little by little. The person alternates between wanting to remain with reality and not, moving away from reality a little at a time without having to make a total commitment. Strokes are a stronger message, often debilitating only on one side of the body as we hover between wanting to stay and wanting to go. But which side is closing down and which side will have to be responsible?

Brain disease is also about not bothering to direct the message to the right place, perhaps because the person feels that it will not be received if the message is sent out. The diseased brain also represents disappointment, of wrong decisions, wrong jobs, wrong partners, wrong life choices.

Those who take drugs, legal and illegal, want to change their reality and do it by changing the brain chemistry. Drug use is a way to deaden the thoughts that are causing pain, a way to retreat into something that will make us feel better, even though the drugs may produce paranoia and fear. But for some people, anything will do to turn off the words that loop around in the brain, and physical illness is related to which words we allowed to loop around.

Words

"I can't think straight," and "my mind is so muddled" are frequently used sayings that state exactly how our thoughts feel—muddled, wobbly and incapable of going in a linear direction. In order to drive a car straight, the wheels have to be in alignment; if not, they pull to one side. Drugs, lack of water or too little nutritious food can also pull the body out of alignment so that the muscles won't work well, the nerves won't spark, and the mind will start to close down.

We say, "My memory is so bad" when we forget things that we think we should remember easily, and the elderly especially talk of having a bad memory. We all have memories we would rather forget, especially if the event was not pleasant, but for the elderly it becomes an excuse not to remember. We forget things close to us when distant memories seem so much better, especially as the end of life approaches.

Forgetfulness often starts when children ask grandparent questions. Not remembering, or not wanting to remember— "I don't remember about that" or "I'm not quite sure"—as the overwhelmed brain cuts in and out, giving the system time to regenerate. People remember at times and not others as gradual weakening of who we are, or the role we have always played, does a slow retreat from life.

The brain is like a muscle and becomes lazy if not used, so if we constantly tell ourselves that we have a bad memory or don't remember, then we are setting in motion the lack of ability to remember. Saying "I forget" when asked about a certain subject suggests a wanting to forget. But what was the incident that needed to be forgotten? Some person or some event? Telling ourselves we are "bored" will also lead to the weakening of the brain's ability to remember, as boredom

The Body's Emotional Imprint

slowly closes down the functioning of the body, too. But boredom is a lack of stimulation and a lack of stimulation produces dull people who live dull, sedentary lives and grow old before their time.

When words become angry and aggressive, those with Alzheimer's usually direct them at some particular action or someone close to them. Often the words are hurtful as they spew "I can do it on my own you stupid woman!" And for those who have lived a good, righteous life, the words can be a stream of swear words,

> George Harrison, referred to as the "quiet" Beatle, died from lung cancer that had metastasized to the brain -- a storehouse of unspoken words. Paul McCartney referred to him as his little brother, but as part of a quartet maybe all he really wanted was an equal voice.

which is a shock for their families but a delight for the one who is finally letting go. We blame the disease for the outburst, but is it really? Do they know what they are saying, but choose to say it anyway? Often these are the people—usually women—who have had to live the "right" life for their parent, spouse or siblings. They keep the charade going until they no longer care, or no longer have the strength to play the game. They approach the end of their lives as the person they have always secretly been: angry, frustrated and disillusioned.

"My brain is so frazzled" indicates an overload, usually from having too much mental work to do, and, "My head hurts," indicates much the same thing. There is information overload with too much coming in and not enough information sent out, and even though we say the words to indicate an overload, most of us don't really listen to the message.

Some now believe that radiation from cell phones is affecting the brain and causing tumors. Constantly talking on the phone causes information to flow in and out and requires the brain to sift through the words to determine what is important and what isn't. If the brain becomes overburdened, then information starts to jam up. We may believe it is the radiation causing the jam/tumor, and it probably is a component, but the fact that some cell phone users grow a tumor and others don't, suggests that some have a more difficult time processing the information—or have trouble with the sound on a cell phone—which is less clear than a landline and requires more effort to hear.

"I could have brained him" usually refers to kids who have the ability to do something, but don't do it. These words are spoken by a frustrated parent about a potentially bright child, but if spoken enough, can lead to a slow eating away and beating down of the child's brain as the words sink in deeper and deeper.

When others talk of wanting to be "very clear about my next move," they can be speaking of an actual move to another home, city or country; or about work, career or a project. It may be a desire to finally get it "right," to clear the mind of unwanted thoughts so that clarity can come through, or to "be clear" to avoid misunderstandings. Even though we may say these words about other situations, it can also represent real clutter at home as the piles of "stuff" stop the flow of thought.

Constantly saying words of being overloaded or unable to think straight is a sign that the brain needs a break. If a break isn't an option, then the brain will slow down and function less and less as it becomes unable to direct the messages to the right place. That's when a nervous breakdown occurs, or dementia begins. We are told that if we keep the mind active, there is less chance of getting Alzheimer's, but an active mind doesn't gather things on a "to do" list. A spry mind takes action. Slow brains have time to dwell on grievances, wanting to get even for all the hurts, humiliations, wrong decisions and other negative words and situations from the past—all dragging along as bottled-up resentment with nowhere to go.

We end up "at my wits end" because a situation or person has put us there. But who or what is driving us to the end of our wits? Wits are usually associated with a keen intelligence, and so losing our wits is serious and implies total exhaustion from thinking too much—perhaps from a demanding situation that requires work, too many family problems, or an overload of financial troubles. As the brain becomes scrambled, so do our problem-solving skills, but perhaps someone else can help. After all "two heads are better than one" if we are willing to ask.

On the other hand, having wit implies someone who is inventive with words and ideas and can use them in a humorous way, as in being a "quick wit." We have a sharp mind when we "use our wits" to move ahead in life. Alzheimer's is about losing the mind slowly and going nowhere.

See Cancer, Right/Left side for additional information.

BREASTS – Cancer

Basic Anatomy

The breasts have mammary glands that provide a baby with milk—a watery, nutrient-laden fluid—during the first few months of its life, and don't become functional until pregnancy occurs. Mammary gland are composed of 15 -20 lobes that radiate out from the nipple. Each lobe is surrounded by fat and connective tissue and divides into smaller lobules which are milk-producing units.

On top of the breast is the areola, a darker circular area that surrounds the nipple, which allows the baby to suckle the milk. The nipples and areolas are connected by a blood supply called the axillary arteries, and the nipples are held erect by smooth muscles that respond to signals from the autonomic nervous system—without conscious effort—to either a cold temperature or to stimulation.

Beneath the tissue of the breast lies the muscle of the chest wall called the pectoralis major muscle. A layer of connective tissue between the two, called fascia, covers all muscle tissue, and linking the breast to the fascia are the ligaments that provide support to the breast. The size of a women's breasts is mostly determined by fatty tissue, but size has no bearing on the amount or the quality of milk produced.

Breasts also contain lymphatic vessels which collect under the arm as lymph nodes and are responsible for protecting the body against infections and disease. This area is where tight bras can bind women's breasts and also the place where deodorants are applied, both of which, some believe, may contribute to breast cancer. Antiperspirants are made from aluminum compounds and parabens—toxic petrochemical derivatives—along with other toxic additives.

Men can also grow breasts, called gynecomastia, although not by choice, as this growth is caused by a chemical imbalance between the levels of the hormones estrogen and testosterone.

Emotional disharmony

Breasts relate to mothering, being a woman, being sexy, being what men want, and what men want women to be. And in this day and age, life has become overwhelming for many women on many levels as they try to be all things to all people. Today, women are expected to be superwomen who can do it all, take care of it all, and be a good mother, wife and a dutiful daughter. And this expectation is taking its toll. Many women delay having children so they can concentrate on their careers, but the delay makes the timing of when to have children that much more difficult as it brings into focus what being female means, what having a job means, and raises if having children will stop them from being attractive, sexy and desirable.

For some women, giving birth signifies the fulfillment of their obligation as a woman. And once that job is finished, it can change the dynamics within a marriage with regard to sexuality, as the focus then shifts to the child and away from the woman and their husband—which is often when marriages break down.

The conflict of career versus children becomes a conflict of being a woman and being torn between two worlds, home and work. Most women love having enlarged breasts while pregnant and breast feeding, but hate the inconvenience of feeding and what it does to their breasts afterwards, so they experience conflicting emotions that can produce miscarriages and other health problems during a pregnancy.

Cancer takes up space in the body crowding out more necessary things, just as time is crowded out with obligations at work and at home, especially as many women have now been forced to take on the male role too, as a single parent. The prevailing belief for breast cancer seem to be one of too much nurturing of others and not enough attention given to the one who is doing the nurturing. But constantly giving to others can lead to resentment, anger, and feeling unappreciated, perhaps by a needy husband, kids, parents, in-laws, or a demanding boss. Anger at having to put a career on hold in order to give birth and do the caregiving, or resentment at having to work, leaving her with little time at home with the baby. Breast cancer is also a reminder of leaving everything to "mother."

Chemotherapy is the way we deal with most cancers as we try to destroy the offending cells, but this also destroys other cells and takes away another part of femininity—hair—and a bald woman, often with a breast removed is not an ideal image of womanhood in our culture. Mastectomies cut away the part of the body that represents female sexuality as the surgery flattens the breasts so they will no longer be noticed. And as only one breast is usually affected, are we cutting away our male, dominant side, or our female side? Is it that we are fed up with men looking at breasts, or that we see breasts as sexual objects that we no longer need? Are we conflicted about wanting to speak our mind but also wanting to be a good girl, or is it that we forbid ourselves to talk about "girly" things in order to work in a man's world? Have we now become our own censor, denying ourselves the pleasures in life?

The Body's Emotional Imprint

Cancer, once it is diagnosed, forces us to rely on others to take care of us. But are we the caretakers out of choice or because we were brought up to believe that we should be out of a sense of duty? Or, is it that we haven't asked for help, and we are afraid that if we did ask, we'd be seen as weak? Or are we afraid that if help did arrive, we would no longer be called a superwoman? Has the need to be a superwoman become a prison of our own choosing?

Many women suffer from swollen breasts before menstruation, but swollen implies that there is too much fluid floating around. Rivers become swollen as the water comes rushing through, just as blood is released during menstruation, which also releases the emotions connected to that blood flow. Blood is red and connected to Cupid and the heart and so, for many women, is an overemotional time as the emotions of self-love flow out. The flow is a reminder that the reason for menstruation is to enable women to give life and a constant message on the to-do list to make a decision to have a child. Or maybe only one partner wants children, causing the menstrual cycle to become a painful reminder of that fact.

Tight bras and underwire bras may also cause breast problems and the decision of which bra to wear is connected to the image a woman wishes to present. Is the bra pushing the breasts up into an unnatural position, or are the breasts allowed to find their own level? Is the image meant to appeal to others or ourselves? Important lymph glands, which are a necessary part of the immune system, are located close to the under arm area, close to where an underwire bra rests.

It's interesting that in the 1960's, as women came out of the kitchens into the workplace, and burned their bras along the way, one of the top models, and the one all young women wanted to emulate, was Twiggy. She was stick thin and had virtually no breasts. Suddenly women didn't care what men thought of their bodies, or about men's opinion on any subject.

In the 1950's, when women were supposed to be virgins before they married and became homemaker and babymaker afterwards, the trend was towards pointed bras stitched in a circular pattern until it came to a point where the nipple was supposed to go. The message to men was "keep away." Today, as women are starting to feel angry at having to fight for abortion and equality all over again, small-chested women are coming back into vogue, as are shorts, short skirts and boots. The message—we can do anything and we don't care what men think.

Words

We can tell a lot by the words we hear others use, and we can also pinpoint what is wrong in a relationship, or what is happening in a society. Even though large numbers of women have been in the work force for over forty years, there are still men who want their women "barefoot and pregnant" and who want their spouse to "smother them with love" once they return home from work. For many women, the response is that they "want to feel free and less burdened" as they see the relationship as unequal since they "carry the weight of the relationship on their shoulders." Others don't want to be seen as a "sex object" and ask "Why doesn't he acknowledge that I have a brain?" while many, ask, "Why am I always the one who has to take care of everything?" or complain that their husband "needs a mother, not a wife." But words have a way of chipping away at our health, little by little, especially if the expectations are not met in a relationship, and this goes for men as well as women. As resentment grows, so does disease.

Many who get cancer and have a mastectomy say to others, "I had it cut away" referring to the breast. But what is actually being cut away, and will it really take away the emotional problem? Did something need to be cut away long before the cancer arrived: a relationship, business, family situation, a money problem? We cut away vegetation when we clear forests that are overgrown, but the same could be said for what we wish to cut back in our own lives: things that now have little meaning, or maybe we feel that we have little meaning in the lives of others. Perhaps children who no longer need us, a spouse who works late, a parent who has recently died.

People say, "It cut him to the quick" when there is a deep wound, and we cut away festering parts of the body when there is little hope of recovery, but if the emotions are left to fester, then the problem will recur. So what really needs to be cut away, and did the surgery complete the task? If not, then what part of the resentment, or unhappiness, remains, and what does it pertain to? And if we cut away a breast thinking it will cut away the problem, but it doesn't, then what body part should we cut away next?

Incidents of breast cancer are higher in developed countries and lower in the less developed ones. Food for thought!

The right breast, representing male attributes, is accepted as the more logical and dominant side, which represents the working environment for many women, so problems on this side can be linked to working in a man's world and not feeling comfortable being there—especially if the men are not supportive. And many women do complain of "not feeling supported" in their work as they struggle against male dominance. But breasts, too, need support, but not with bras that are so tight that they bind them. Sometimes men don't support women in a workplace because the women are too aggressive, too sexy, too much of a threat to their manhood, or their job. Even women working with other women often feel unsupported and compelled to "hold their own" against them.

The left breast represents the need to acquiesce to superiors, often leading to feeling belittled by the experience, which over time, will lead to sickness or cancer. How we respond to the men in our lives can cause us to overcome problems or feel defeated by a society that constantly devalues women. In the west—especially in American culture—the breasts are an important part of sexuality, which is why many women, especially celebrities, feel the need to show them off to prove their worth. Big breasts, bigger paycheck. Age can also be a factor in illness, as we ask "Does this make me look old?" and the fear and dread of being "too old for the job."

A philandering husband can also make us feel less desirable. But if he's the one philandering, why do we take it out on our own body and not on him?—unless we think that making ourselves sick will bring him back, will make him pay attention, make him feel guilty, and "make him pay the price"?

Illness often shows up when we need to prove how valuable we are. Women who have cancer often ask their family, "How are you going to cope without me?" as if others are incapable of running the home. But is the family the problem, or our need to control? At other times we want to "make a clean breast of it" in order to feel better, which is probably why some breast lumps disappear instead of becoming cancerous. What we think, we manifest.

We live in a body-conscious culture, and very rarely are women satisfied with their breast size, but if women were, would we have such a high incidence of breast cancer?

See Chest and Lymphatic system for additional information

BRUISES – Abuse

Basic Anatomy

Bruising, also called contusion, is caused by a blow or pressure and occurs when the skin is not broken but the tissue underlying the skin becomes injured. When the small blood vessels rupture, the blood drains into the surrounding area, resulting in swelling and "black and blue" marks. It usually takes several days for a bruise to begin the healing process, going from a reddish color to dark blue and finally to a yellowish brown as the color slowly fades away as the blood under the skin is absorbed back into the surrounding tissue.

Bruising can also occur spontaneously in the elderly, especially women, when over time, the tissues supporting the capillaries weaken and become more fragile and prone to rupture.

Thinning skin is another reason why the elderly bruise more easily, as the protective fatty layer that helps cushion the blood vessels against injury, begins to weaken. Arms and legs are typical locations for bruises—appendages that we use the most—although bruises can also appear over the entire body.

Emotional disharmony

Bruising is not as serious as other illnesses and accidents, but nevertheless is an unsaid cry for help, especially from the elderly who are prone to bruising from lack of good nutrition or from falls or knocking into objects as their balance becomes less stable. Lack of desire to prepare healthy meals, or lack of money to buy fresh produce, is a problem for many elderly and bruises are outward signs that all is not well and they need some support in their lives. How big and discolored the bruising area is, is an indication of how deeply they need emotional or physical help.

Bruising isn't as harsh as a broken bone or a sprain and doesn't stop our motion, but it does affects our outer shell, the skin, which is the link between our inner and outer worlds. It is our protective covering, which when bruised, shows discoloration and disfigurement that allows the world to see just how hurt we really are as the emotions project from the inside out.

Those infected with HIV/AIDS, bruise easily, as the immune system and blood supply—our life force—slowly drains away, although not everyone with the infection dies, so those who continue on have found a way of making themselves strong enough to withstand the bruising of an uncaring world—or a series of uncaring partners.

Young children bruise easily from a lack of understanding of time, space or objects, and because they are unable to withstand the physical or verbal bruising inflicted on them by others, or by change in their lives that they are unable to cope with. Always in a hurry, they trip over their own feet to get to something, someone or some place. But are they running from something or to something? Is the mind running quicker than the feet, leaving them with things they want to accomplish but without the physical means to do so, or are they running from an abusive situation?

Children and the elderly who are physically abused, often receive bruises where they can't be seen: on the legs and the torso and places covered with clothing. The marks are hidden from view, leaving the one who inflicted the bruise able to get away with the action but leaving the one who is bruised to live with the emotional marks long after the discoloration has disappeared.

Where bruising takes place is an indication of what emotions are being played out. Eyes are especially susceptible as we fall into objects that we don't see, or we don't want to see who has caused the emotional or physical bruise. Legs and arms move forward, backwards and outwards, and so bruising here shows that the forward movement isn't sound or that someone is stopping an action from taking place. It can also indicate that going backwards isn't the movement we want to make, referring perhaps to a demotion at work, moving back with parents we thought we had left forever or with an ex-spouse who won't leave us alone. If we receive a bruise from being in too much of a hurry but are unafraid to move forwards, no matter what obstacles are placed in our way, then we may be moving too quickly and need to step back to review the situation more closely.

The blood supply which forms the initial bruise takes time to be reabsorbed back into the body, leaving us time to reflect on the cause of a fall/accident. Do we need to slow down? Are we driving ourselves too hard and it is wearing us down? We make the excuse that we walked or tripped into something, but the bruising indicates that we are not feeling secure in our surroundings. But where are the surroundings, at work or home?

Did an accident occur in relation to some form of transportation? Are we upset at having to travel so far to work? To take an action that we don't want to take? Are we stumbling because we are not feeling supported in a relationship or a work environment? Where the falling takes place indicates how strong we feel in that environment, and as many elderly people fall outside their home, it shows how unsafe they feel outside where they have to navigate people and situations.

Getting into a fight often produces bruising and is also a sign that all is not well and help is needed to sort through the aggression to stop future outbreaks. It may be an outward discoloration on the skin, but it really reflects an inner emotion that is asking for help. But which side are we on, the one doing the bruising or the one receiving it? Do we need help to stop the aggressive person from bruising others? Does the bruise, in a way, replace words that should have been spoken? Do we need to talk through the problem, and are both sides willing to talk—or is it a one-sided fight?

If bruising is a regular occurrence and is usually in the same place on the body, then what recurring issue do we need to take care of? What problem are we refusing to deal with: is it medical, financial, or, related to family? Do we want to relocate but are too timid to make the break from a job, location, marriage? Are we looking ahead to anticipate the future, but not taking care of the present?

Words

Bruises are about being hurt emotionally, and the type of hurt we are receiving, or giving to others. Very often we dismiss the bruise as inconsequential, as the skin isn't damaged and no bones were broken, but then we also dismiss the emotional connection too.

We talk of "bruised egos" and of having our "feelings bruised" when the things we hold most dear to us are damaged. But who is doing the bruising? Are we doing it to ourselves as punishment for something we feel guilty about? Or are we allowing others to perform the task? Women often stay in abusive relationships and endure the violence by believing they deserved to be hit, either for something they didn't do or for something they did do, but really staying in the relationship is a cry to be loved, even by an abusive partner. The love which occurs when making up is the coming together of two needy, emotionally bruised, beings.

> In an emergency, frozen vegetables make a great cold pack to apply to a bruise. Unfortunately, once defrosted you then have to eat them -- unless they are vegetables you really dislike, in which case refreeze them ready for the next bruise.

Men, especially, who "give a real bruiser" are really angry at themselves for not being better or attaining more in life, or for not being the person they wish they were, and often behave violently to force the one receiving the bruising to leave them. The subconscious goes very deep, and feeling that we are worthless and unlovable can cause us to do things against another that we wouldn't normally do. Verbal abuse works the same way, as we push out those most needed in our lives. Men who are unable to find the words to express their feelings are often the perpetrators of violence. A need to show who's the boss. No bones are broken but the mark on the skin serves as one-upmanship, puncturing the outer, protective layer. Violence is a way to send a message without words.

A bruise also goes through a color transaction, from dark to light, passing through yellow, indicating that he was "yellow," or cowardly and lacked the guts to fight back. The guy was "cruisin for a bruisin" and next time may "get it." Men usually speak of such actions to threaten other men and for bravado. Unable to provide for a family economically, they can provide protection in the form of violence.

We often say, "I felt black and blue from the argument" to express how we feel as we are figuratively beaten up by a boss, spouse, or others, while we say, "I felt as if I'd been hit by a truck" to show that the body and mind can't take on any more abuse. Very often these words are unspoken, but the bruises on the body shows that there is a problem and it needs attention.

The color blue is also connected to "feeling blue," or depressed, and when the color becomes even darker, as in "a black mood," then the mood can't get any darker and the need for help from others has increased. An unpredictable boss or spouse who is in a "black mood" can cast a pall of fear over the entire environment, and anyone working under these conditions will eventually become stressed and tired. We refer to these people as casting a "dark cloud" over the place as the mood drags everyone down with them. And giving someone a "black eye" is to give them a "real shiner," and implies a punch that was supposed to put an end to what-ever the problem was—and whoever was causing it. Black is not a happy color and in the west is connected to funerals and the end of life.

Bruising is also connected to blood in cases of anemia, when people feel "completely drained" and have nothing left to give as they run out of everything life-giving. We "give" bruises to others and we "receive a bruising" as if we were receiving a gift, which it can be if we accept it as a wake-up call that we need to change something. So what do we need to learn from a bruising? Do we need to change to a more secure location, relationship or workplace?

"I tripped and fell," when spoken by the elderly, is often an excuse for muscle weakness or a problem with balance, but it also shows a fear of being alone. If the fall is inside the home, then they are lonely and need outside intervention. If they fall outside the home, then they feel insecure and would feel much more protected if they had someone to walk with them to do their shopping, and go to doctor's appointments and other outings. They may never ask for the help, but the fall is their plea. When the elderly have many falls, it is a cry for help as they start to feel frail and see the end in sight. And a series of small falls will very often lead to bigger ones as they see death approaching, however, if they are given the support and attention they need, many elderly can have a "new lease on life" and go on for many more years.

See applicable Body sections for additional information.

CHEST – Ribcage

Basic Anatomy

The chest is the front region of the body between the neck and the abdomen and encases the most important organs of the body: the heart, lungs and liver. The ribcage is part of the chest, the bony structure that the chest is built on and around, connecting the front to the spine.

The sternum, a flat, elongated, bone that runs down the front from the throat and separates the two sets of ribs, is about seven inches long and protects the heart, lungs and major blood vessels.

The rib cage consists of 24 ribs, twelve on each side. The first seven, called the true ribs, are connected directly to the sternum by cartilage, flexible connective tissue that allows for the elasticity of the ribcage as the lungs expand and contract for efficient breathing. The next three ribs are called the false ribs and connect to the sternum via additional cartilage attached to the ribs above, while the last 2 ribs are considered floating ribs as they attach only to the vertebrae of the spinal column and have no attachment to the sternum at the front.

Holding it all together is a complex system of muscles that crisscross around the side of the ribcage to connect the chest to the spine, and other muscles that attach the shoulders and arms to the chest and neck.

Emotional disharmony

Men often puff out their chests in the company of other men as a way to try and look aggressive, threatening, or in control of a situation. It is a form of one-upmanship, although, usually there is another male ready to deflated the first one's chest by a physical or verbal blow, to send a message that the chest was puffed out too far. On the other hand, it can be a mating call to women, a way of preening, much like birds do.

People who need to deflect anger or verbal abuse will cover the chest area, crossing the arms over the chest in a protective manner. As the arms cross over, the back becomes more rounded as a way of going within and remaining safe under a protective shell, not wanting to show vulnerability. Women cross their arms over the chest, one hand holding the alternate arm/elbow, as a protective measure to cover their breasts, often from others staring at them, or to ward off hurtful words, or to keep others from becoming too close—often in the company of men or those in authority. Men, on the other hand, usually cross their arms as a sign of strength and authority reflecting a different interpretation of what the chest signifies.

The chest is a protective covering that totally envelopes the upper part of the body, where the most important vital organs are located. Broken bones in the chest/rib area suggests a weakness of that protective layer, and a vulnerability in the most important organs; the heart, liver and lungs. All three organs are vital for life, so where the bones are broken will indicate which organ is the most vulnerable. The sternum, the broad central bone, protects the heart from damage, and the ribcage protects the lungs and most of the liver. Broken or cracked ribs or sternum can take many months to heal, a painful process as each breath taken pushes against the bones, reminding us of the vulnerability and frailty of the body and also the cause of the damage.

Usually, ribs are broken from an accident or sports injury, so it's important to think about what was happening before the injury occurred. Do we really want to play the sport we were injured in? Was it a car accident, and if so, who was at the wheel? Was the trip to somewhere unpleasant or a return trip from an unpleasant experience? Who or what was involved? Was the break into two pieces or a complete shattering of the ribs?

The strength of the bones of the ribcage reflects how strong we feel our protective armor is, and how safe the organs behind the ribs are. Would the ribcage protect us from a fatal fall, crash, or from something we deem stronger than ourselves? Cracked or bruised ribs also indicate a feeling of insecurity regarding what we have gathered around us: family, money, possessions, health. We often have accidents when we are not paying attention, but the reason behind the inattention could be a money problem, or worry about some future event.

Any problem with the ribs is serious, not just because the ribcage is hurt, but also because it implies that the barrier that protects the most important organs has been breached, much like the wall of a castle protecting the people behind it, and so it requires serious thought as to why the injury occurred. Does the ribcage give us enough room for our lungs to breathe, or are they being pushed inwards by our posture? If the posture becomes too constricted, then it will also affect the workings of the heart, lungs and stomach.

We exercise our backs muscles thinking it will give us flexibility, but without expanding the chest muscles too, the entire chest will pull inwards as the back muscles become much broader and stronger than the front ones. We need balance in our lives so that we can weather whatever life throws at us, but if some muscles are not given the freedom to stretch, then, eventually, they will shorten and the entire torso will deform.

Open heart surgery is much less invasive nowadays, but for years it entailed the cutting open of the ribs with a saw and then prizing them apart in order to get to the heart to perform the surgery. It's a traumatic experience for every part of the body: blood, bones, muscles and emotions, and one that imprints on every cell in the body. Very often people who have had open heart surgery that require the ribs to be cut, complain of tiredness afterwards; sometimes for months and sometimes for the rest of their lives. But is the tiredness from the surgery or the emotional trauma that was inflicted on the body? And what emotions did the surgery bring up—anger, humiliation, love, fear? Cutting into the ribs also exposes the vulnerability of the heart and all the emotions stored there. Just as the ribcage can guard against attacks, so also it can stop love from entering. Heart surgery is often a chance for that to change, allowing love to enter or allowing the person to become a more loving person.

Words
We relate the chest to the need to get something "off our chest" whether it's words, people or situations. The weight is squeezing the life out of us, and we need to get rid of the circumstances causing the problem, perhaps money worries, a job that is no longer satisfying, words that need to be spoken to others. Most of these words related to the chest suggest something or someone who has really damaged us, and in some cases, so severely that the organs behind the ribs have also been damaged. Hearing others talk of "getting

The Body's Emotional Imprint

something off my chest" or "I feel as if I have a crushing weight on my chest," suggests a deep worry that could become a serious health problem if not dealt with. It could also imply guilt that is so intense that it needs to be expressed before it affects the emotional health.

The chest has a different meaning for men than for women. A large chest for a man signifies manliness, especially if it is accompanied with slim hips, which suggest a man who is toned, rugged, adventurous, and a "real" man. These men equate the chest with sexuality as they "puff out their chests," usually with their legs placed wide apart as a way of taking up space and "marking their territory." The word "chest" for women refers to the body that lies under the breasts. The breasts are sexual and important, while what lies beneath is secondary.

> Words follow fashion and when tightly laced corsets were worn, it forced women to breathe from the upper portion of their lungs, hence the term "heaving bosoms."

When we talk of those who "can't take a ribbing," we mean someone who can't take a joke; this is usually said to protect the one making the statement, who knows it really is no joke. Often said in a malicious manner, it is a way of saying something cruel but making a joke out of it to protect themselves. Verbally abusive people often say this as a way of humiliating others in such a sly way that they cannot be faulted. On the other hand, "I laughed until my ribs hurt" could reflect either genuine amusement, or laughter at another's expense.

We speak of "receiving a crushing blow" when the severe blow has reaches through the ribcage to the vital organs. Crushing blows wind us and "knock the stuffing out of us," which suggests that the lungs were damaged, making it difficult to breathe. "It knocked the wind out of my sails" also describes a blow so forceful that the shock "left me speechless." Many times, we are "taken off guard" by others saying hurtful and unexpected words that leave us unable to respond. We "let our guard down" much like a boxer who didn't protect himself against the final "crushing blow" that ended the fight. Just as the hurtful words will probably end the relationship with another.

If we repeat these words over and over again, then the crushing blow that has affected us so deeply could link back to a devastating emotional blow from which the body may never recover—a family death, illness, economic situation or character assassination. Breathing is difficult, all love has gone—and the heart, lungs and liver are all damaged. We may "try to put on a good front" like a Hollywood movie set, but the inside is hurting.

When we feel good about our position in life, we stand erect so that the underlying organs can perform freely. We look strong and feel strong.

See Heart, Liver, Lungs for additional information.

COLON – Large Intestine

Basic Anatomy

The colon, also called the large intestine, is attached to the small intestine and moves waste material through to the rectum, absorbing water, salts and some nutrients from the mass before forming it into stools for elimination. About 5 feet in length, it divides into three main area: the ascending colon, which winds upwards on the right side of the body; the transverse colon, which continues across the top of the abdomen under the stomach and liver, and the descending colon, which travels down the left side of the abdomen. From there it continues into a very short curve known as the sigmoid colon and then enters the rectum, the final eliminating point.

The colon has no real digestive function, but the muscles that line the walls work to reabsorb liquid from the mass in order to recycle it back into the body before squeezing the contents along in a wave movement to the rectum. Billions of beneficial bacteria, called flora, coat the colon to provide a healthy balance within the body and to prevent the proliferation of harmful bacteria.

A misshapen colon is often caused by a buildup of fecal matter on the walls, often from too little liquid, which allows parasites to proliferate, causing gas and bloating. This buildup can take place over months or even years as the fecal matter hardens into a cement-like mass. As more and more waste builds up, the opening of the intestines become smaller and smaller, making it difficult to eliminate the waste and causing the matter to stay in the intestines for a longer period of time.

A prolapsed transverse colon can result in pressure on the small intestines and, in women, on the uterus below. This can cause pain and menstrual cramps, and also urinary incontinence if the pressure affects the bladder.

A healthy colon should produce 2-3 bowel movements a day.

Emotional disharmony

The colon represents how well we process our lives and how well we are able to take out whatever nourishment—internally and externally—we need along the way to support a healthy system. If we are not nourished, or perceive that we were not given enough support and love when young, or were not able to accept it when it was offered, then eventually a blockage will appear in the colon that will stop the normal flow of waste, and of emotions.

This is where we may form a barrier against the love from others and the enjoyment of life, choosing instead to allow a buildup of negativity that refuses to move on and out. The obstruction can come from too many possessions that require time, too much work, too many things to care for, too many people to take care of, too many papers and legal obligations, or just being unable to say or do anything to remover the emotional load. We may feel responsible but hate every moment of it, want to be free, but know that it isn't possible, or want to dislodge the resentment, but know it has grown too large to move. Colons are like rivers that deposit sediment at the end of their journey. Everything is fine while the water is running freely, but problems arise when the sediment is ignored and silt builds up.

When we are burdened, stressed or constantly interrupted, traveling for business, or have too many clients to meet with too many lunches and dinners in restaurants, then regular bowel movements become difficult, making the waste back up instead of releasing it when the body needs to. The colon is where the remains of meals pass through and out, so if there is a blockage, where in the colon is it? Is the obstruction recent, as at the beginning and giving us time to deal with it, in the middle which is much harder to reach, or the end, where it refuses to move out?

The ascending colon, on the right of the body, represents the more male, dominant side, the descending colon, on the left, represents the female side; these sides are connected by the transverse colon. So which side is the problem? Or maybe the problem lies in the middle, as we alternate between what we want versus what others expect from us. Should we follow our own path or the path others have chosen for us? The battle can also be between our male and female traits.

Colon cancer, which has become more prevalent today, is based on sadness that has built up over the years and has turned into resentment of things not said, resentment of others, and resentment of a life that hasn't played out as expected. Unable to move, the cancer grows until we no longer have the ability to do the things we wanted to do or live the life we wanted to live, or become the person we always imagined we would become. Holding onto the problem for too long and not having the will to act on it when we should have, we turn the anger and resentment back on the body to let it devour itself. Unable to process life any longer and deal with the disappointments and responsibilities, many with the disease give up as their support system slowly falls away, leaving the cancer to eventually take life away too.

The transverse colon, which passes beneath the stomach, is the segment that can become prolapsed, a condition where the colon droops down, pushing onto the organs below it. Food that remains in there too long could be the cause, as can lack of muscles strength, which is connected to feeling weak emotionally. As the prolapsed colon drops down onto other organs, it may eventually push the uterus down too, causing us to see that as the problem, rather than the prolapsed colon. The transverse colon also links the two sides, right and left, male and female, so there could be a division in the family, marriage, workplace, or a conflict about the direction we want to take—the more creative side or the more logical side. The responsibility of trying to reconcile the two sides may be the reason for our colon problem.

Polyps of the colon are growths of extra tissue inside the walls, so what small irritations have we allowing to grow in there? Small things that we have interpreted as big ones. What irritating person or event have we allowed to antagonize us? Polyps aren't a complete blockage but they are an obstacle course for matter/emotions to pass through, so who is making us jump through hoops? Any kind of restriction in the colon is a blockage of negative thoughts that we have allowed to accumulate, forcing their release through surgery.

Colitis is a chronic inflammation of the colon, and anything inflamed is hot, indicating an unexpressed anger. Inflammation also burns up the cells that line the colon, opening the door to bacteria that can cause festering and soreness. A sore is painful and can result from a repetitive action such as a rubbing motion, but in the case of the colon, the friction is internal and has built up into a fire. If bacteria has entered, then the defenses are down and we feel weak against invaders, who could be someone who will not move out of our

The Body's Emotional Imprint

home or leave us alone, or a situation we cannot avoid, such as a family member who constantly make demands on us. If we refuse to talk about the problem because it has become a "sore point" then it is definitely time to address the issue—before it becomes a serious wound. Sometimes wounds don't heal and produce an open lesion—one which is on show for everyone to see, so is there someone we are hoping to humiliate in public, an ex-spouse perhaps? And is that person really worth that much aggravation and illness?

Words

There are so many places in the colon for blockages to occur that it's amazing anything passes through it. But even if we don't know we have a conspicuous obstruction, our bodies will tell us by word such as "I just can't seem to get past this" or "I just can't let it go." The distress we feel from holding on to a problem is causing pain and illness.

We say, "He put up barriers that stopped me from doing my job" about a person who makes life difficult for others. But often the blockage is in the colon of the people holding back the words because they don't want to say anything confrontational to the offending person, leaving the colon to bear the brunt.

We erect barriers to stop others from invading our territory, and we erect emotional barriers to stop the words of others, but barriers also stop things from flowing through, which then becomes a one sided argument, deal or agreement benefiting the opposition. So what are we allowing to build up that is causing us, but not the offending party, pain? Anger, resentment, hostility? Is there a tactful way to lift the barrier? Is there a way to talk through the problem or some way around it?

We often talk of others who "blocked my progress," but maybe our response to them formed the barrier in the first place. If we take the barrier down—by seeing their side of things—then maybe the colon problem will subside too.

> Even though the large intestine is much shorter than the small intestine, the circumference is larger than the small intestine, hence the names.

"I'm burning mad" can be related to colitis if the colon is inflamed. But who or what is fanning the flames? Something or someone that can be controlled, doused, put out? Smoldering embers eventually erupt into fires, so find the trigger point before that happens and deal with it—and find who or what keeps pressing that trigger point.

A fire suggests a rage, which can go beyond health issues into a rage when driving, a rage at work, or a rage at a loved one. People who are full of rage are frightening to others as fires erupt and can become difficult to dampen, and erupting people are unsettling. If we constantly have to gauge how someone else will respond to whatever we say, then eventually we become guarded in our speech. Guarded speech leads to secrets, lack of accountability and a slow decline, whether in a marriage, business or government relationship. If the rage comes from someone else—a boss or spouse—who won't get help, then find a way to leave. Uncontrollable rage is destructive and ruins lives and families.

Diverticulitis occurs when feces become trapped in pouches that have formed along the intestine walls, allowing bacteria to grow and cause an infection. If the immune system is not strong enough to overcome the infection, we may feel as if we are being "eaten away." These words suggests that someone is attacking us slowly and methodically. Verbal abuse affects us in different ways and in different parts of our body, and if we are unable to fight back with words because the other person is stronger or in a higher position, then the colon can become a dumping ground for the pent-up anger as the words mount up. Small outbursts of anger send words outwards, which may affect the sender or the receiver. But who is the outburst directed at, and why? And is the right person receiving it or should it be directed towards another? Bullies attack others at their most vulnerable and bacteria do the same thing.

The words "I feel as if everything in my life has collapsed" could relate to the colon becoming weakened from overeating and a constant backup of food that isn't processed in a timely manner, or to muscles that have weakened the colon's ability to function well. We may be battling on, but, through these words, the body is telling us otherwise.

When we have colon problems, saying "This job is killing me" is the body's way of giving us a choice between either the job or health. What are we willing to give up and what are we willing to endure in order to make a living? And if someone has "opened a festering wound," then it pertains to something internal that is festering, such as a relationship that won't allow us to move on.

See Bowels, Stomach and Uterus for additional information.

CUTS

Basic Anatomy

Cuts are open wounds that separate the connective tissue in the skin. They can be deep or superficial, but the deeper they go, the more painful they become and the more bacteria are able to enter the wound. Sharp object such as knives or shards of glass cause most cuts, but if the cut is very deep, then we refer to it as a gash, which usually requires stitches and can produce a scarring of the tissue. Broken skin can also occur from animal or human bites, often causing an infection that requires medical attention.

The outer layer of skin, called the epidermis, contains nerves but no blood vessels, but as a cut goes deeper, through layers of fat, connective tissue, blood vessels, nerve endings and sweat glands, so a cut becomes more dangerous, especially when it goes down to the underlying bones and organs.

Cuts over joints usually take longer to heal as movement can constantly reopen the wound, while cuts that go down to the bone can infect the bone itself. Injuries that remove the tip of a finger will often result in nerve damage and loss of sensation at the tip, and open wounds to the head and face bleed more than wounds to other parts of the body as they have a large blood supply closer to the surface.

The body begins to repair a wound immediately, but while some people have quick-healing skin, others take much longer to heal depending on their immune system's response, general health and age, the type of cut and whether or not it has become infected.

The Body's Emotional Imprint

People who have had limbs removed can experience phantom limb sensations such as severe pain, tingling, cramping or temperature changes in the portion where the limb was removed. The limb may be gone, but the nerve endings at the site are still sending signals to the brain that the limb is still there. Within a few months the sensations decrease, and for most people they will disappear entirely,

When a cut occurs, the damaged tissue causes platelets to clump together around the cut. Chemicals and proteins are then released to form plasma, which is a blood-clotting substance necessary to stop bleeding. The faster attention is paid to the injury—cleaning the wound, stopping the bleeding and closing the cut—the lower the risk of infection.

Emotional disharmony

Cuts imply a desire to self-mutilate, which some do on purpose, but where the cut is on the body will point to what our thoughts are, or were, before the cut occurred. Very often cuts are on our exposed body parts, the face, hands or feet.

Men often cut themselves while shaving, which is a nick to the external appearance as thoughts wander while looking at their face in the mirror. But what are the thoughts about? Liking the image, or finding fault, not only with the image, but with who they are deeper under the skin layers? Or maybe the cut was really directed at someone else, or based on a resistance to shaving to conform to society's standards.

Hands and fingers are things we use constantly, appendages that most of us need in order to function on a daily basis. How we use our hands and fingers before we cut them often shows how we are feeling about the action, or about the location where the action is taking place. Cuts usually occur around knives, scissors and tools, but it's the emotional connection to the object that causes the cut: chopping food, cutting meat when we are vegetarian, cutting out a project that we didn't want to do, or resenting helping someone in their home. Will the cut stop us from continuing the action, or is it a slight cut that will just delay it?. Or are we trying to do something that is too difficult for us? Many children cut themselves when using scissors because they are still unaccustomed to using sharp instruments. They want to do it, but lack the dexterity. So what are we doing that may be the wrong action to take at this point?

The feet are related to our movement forward, and although cuts won't halt us, they can make walking difficult and painful. Cuts can occur when we step on a sharp object or when we engage in a sports activity, so are we doing something we don't want to do in a place we don't want to be in, with the person we don't want to be with? Is the cut going to stop us from moving forward, or stop us from attending an event we don't want to attend?

A cut is a quick action which results in a slowing down of what we were doing, a recognition that our concentration wandered, or we were too distracted to pay attention to the job at hand—or just didn't want to do it at all. Cuts can be deep or shallow, require stitches or just a bandage, but they always require attention—a time out, or time for someone to acknowledge us. They also draw blood and red is the color of life, so is life draining away from us? Do we need a change or an ending to some difficult situation?

People who use electric saws often nip the tops off their fingers from a lack of attention, or from being too familiar and too sure that they are in control of the machine. But the

The Body's Emotional Imprint

inattention and the lost finger part suggests that the project may have been wrong, or the client was the wrong fit, or there is resentment toward the person who commissioned the project.

Sometimes we allow others to cut into us, as in surgery, which cuts into various parts of the body, especially the knee, hip, foot, spine, hand and shoulder, but what problem is the surgery really fixing? What have we avoided doing that now requires someone else to fix the problem by cutting and invading the skin? What emotions have we avoided?

Cutting into the skin produces blood as it goes beyond the surface, just as we must go deeper to explain the reason for the cut. What do we need to pay attention to before it results in some disfigurement? Are we trying to cut away a problem or the person who caused it? Is the cut really an accident or did we we misjudged the situation?

We don't acknowledge things we don't value, so look at the body part that has been cut. The body often directs our attention to a bigger emotional problem that is not being fully dealt with. Hands allow us to perform many tasks, but once cut, they need time to heal, so we may be trying to achieve too much too soon. We cut into flesh and the blood releases the emotions, but how deep is the cut? Depressed people sometimes attempt suicide by slitting their wrists, the area where many veins congregate, making the blood drain out faster to speed up the process of dying. But it is usually a cry for a release from circumstances that have become unbearable, a need to cut away the emotional pain.

Cuts and accidents often suggest an ambivalence about a situation we are about to move into—marriage, a job we are not sure is the right choice, a new location where we are of two minds—just as the mind wanders before the accident happens.

The act of cutting is done to remove something that is unnecessary, unsightly or something that doesn't belong. It is a quick action and usually irreversible, and in emotional terms it represents a deep hurt, not something life-threatening such as organ failure, but a problem that requires action. Even a superficial scratch can draw blood, but blood carries oxygen around the body and oxygen gives us life, so any blood that is lost signifies lost life support, which may be the real reason for the wound.

Words

Cuts are usually quick and short, with little pain until the blood flows, then the ache begins, not from actual pain, but from the sight of blood. Cuts make us pay attention as we utter the words "I didn't pay attention to the job at hand," which suggests that we didn't feel the need to pay attention before the cutting. So what have we started that needs attention before it blows into something much bigger? What problem is small now, but could become full-blown later? Where does the cut indicate the problem lies and what body part is being affected?

Cutting is an absolute action with no wavering. We often say, "I cut him/her off," about offspring' and other family members who have done something so unforgivable that they have been stripped of any right to be included in family gatherings or ventures. Cuts are usually permanent, which is why many say "I've cut them out of my will" or "cut their inheritance." A cutting action is deep, long lasting—often leaving a scar—and is usually in response to a terrible action or words. Often, the one cut off will say in response, "I was cut to pieces," meaning they were devastated about the outcome, which, now that the inheritance has been "cut," will automatically "cut them down to size." The cutting action in a family, business or divorce is often permanent and volatile. If a limb is cut off, then the action is irreversible. It will never grow back and the relationship has been severed for good, which is why many family members never reunite.

Elderly people often talk about "cutting him/her out of my will," as whoever is being cut goes out of favor. Feeling vulnerable, the elderly want to feel needed and loved for who they are, but become angry and afraid if they are not—especially by family and close friends. Feeling disappointed by the family, they "cut back" on gifts to them and see money as the only thing they have as a weapon to bring people into their lives—or not to let them leave in the first place. Saying

> Before a congressional hearing, the subcommittee chairman said that he expected Tony Hayward, of the Gulf of Mexico oil spill, to be "spliced and diced" by both himself and other members. Obviously, Hayward just "wasn't cut out for the job."

they "cut me to the quick" implies a deeper emotional hurt that won't heal quickly. "I'm all cut up about it," indicates the same thing: the emotional impact is very deeply felt on every level as it cuts through to the inner layers, causing pain.

When we turn the words on ourselves, they become just as deep, just as scarring, and just as long-lasting, as we belittle ourselves in front of others. The lack of self-worth shows as an invisible scarring of who we are. Sometimes the scarring comes from childhood when we were "cut down" verbally by an overbearing parent, and other times from domineering family members who feel the need to "cut us to the quick." The quick is soft, tender flesh, usually under the nails, so obviously they want to get under our skin. They feel terrible about who they are, and they are determined to make us feel the same.

"I want to draw blood" indicates a violent act against another, the blood indicating that the wound is significant. We also talk of "seeing red" when we are angry, which implies the desire to draw blood from another, just as wild animals "draw blood" when they attack. We say, "I haven't even scratched the surface" when we haven't finished something. Scratching doesn't break the skin, unless we keep scratching, but it will cause an irritation—meaning that we won't "let the subject die."

Money and the word "cut" often go together, as money frequently has a negative connotation. We give someone a "cut of money" from jobs done, but "cut them out" if we decide not to give them anything. When a job is "cut," it is the "unkindest cut of all." The action taken is swift and decisive and the person who has lost their job feels the loss deeply as it "wounds" the self-esteem and -confidence.

Someone who is "a cut above the rest" is superior, and no one else can match their quality, but someone who wasn't "cut out for the mission" is on the opposite end of the scale. We verbally "cut people down to size" when we want to show who's the boss. Very often the verbal cutting is all that's available and is punishment for something that we have little control over.

When driving, we often "cut people off" by not allowing another into our space. The "cutting off" is usually done to stop their action and to make them know they "have been cut." If a relationship needs ending, we often "cut it off" so that it really ends and can't restart, but if we cut ourselves in the process, then the action of "cutting the cord" on the other person is often something we may regret later. It's a self-mutilation to make us remember that even though we may not be able to live with the person, we also may still not be able to let them go permanently. It's important to see who is doing the cutting and who receives the cut, and also to remember that a cut is a deep, swift penetration of our outer covering; the one we show to the world—and it will leave a mark on us as a reminder of the event.

See Skin and body parts affected for additional information.

EARS – Hearing

Basic Anatomy

Ears are part of the auditory system and are composed of the outer ear, the middle ear and the inner ear, with each part performing an important function in the process of hearing and balance; the first two for hearing, the inner ear for balance.

Hearing occurs as sound enters the ear canal and sets in motion the vibration of the eardrum and middle ear bones. Sound travels as a wave and then activates the hair cells, which convert the energy of sound into a nerve impulse so that it can be understood by the brain.

The outer ear which is called the pinna—the visible ear lobe— collects and localizes the direction of the sound and also protects the ear drum from damage. Sweat glands inside the ear canal, form ear wax for the protection of the inner ear.

The middle ear is an air-filled space in the bone of the skull that sends sound waves through the ear canal to hit the tympanic membrane, which as the name implies, is the ear drum. The middle ear also equalizes air pressure via the tube called the Eustachian tube, which is connected to the back of the nose and is responsible for the "popping" in the ears when there is a change in altitude.

The inner ear is a delicate warren of fluid-filled canals, encased in the skull. At the rear are three liquid-filled loops, called semicircular canals, which send nerve messages to the brain to signal a change in head position so that the muscles can maintain balance. At the front of the inner ear is the cochlea, which resembles a snail' shell and is lined with tiny hairs. When the vibrations—sound—reach the cochlea, the hairs move and translate the vibrations into nerve messages via the auditory nerve, and then travel as impulses to the brain in order for it to understand the information.

Emotional disharmony

How good our hearing is depends on how much we want to hear and how much importance we place on what we are hearing. But even if we are able to hear clearly, if the words are not those we wish to acknowledge then "selective" hearing often comes into play, especially among the elderly and children. We close people out when they dominate the conversation and are boring or if their ideas are incompatible with our own.

Many young children have ear infections, but this could be caused more from words they don't understand or wish to close out, than an ear infection. How many of them hear parents arguing, family members shouting, words that pertain to themselves or to a relative's health, or words at school from a bully or critical teacher? Ear infections are a means of defense when children feel defenseless. Earache is connected to words that make the ears ache, critical words about ourselves or others that we love. Hearing hurtful words about others can affect us just as much as hearing hurtful words about ourselves. An ache is less painful than a hurt, but can go on for a longer period of time.

Hearing problem usually affect one ear more than the other, so it's important to see which ear is most affected. Harsh words from a mother, sister, wife or coworker, may make us more defensive on the left side, while those spoken by the males at home or work may affect the opposite side. Which parent is doing the attacking and which one is on the receiving end? If the words are coming from the father and are hurtful to the mother, then we may block out the female side so that the words can't reach their destination. Or it may be the other way around, with the father being verbally attacked and we need to close down the words from the mother.

The same applies to any relationship, especially for the elderly who have sons and daughters who want to put them into a home. Is it the son or daughter who is doing the pushing? Is one making the demands and closing down the voice of the other side? Most of us don't think about which ear we use, but maybe if we did, it would give us a clearer idea of the emotional involvement.

In other cases, family member may have passed on, but the words still linger in the ears as the hurtful words are replayed over and over again. Many adults who have had hearing problems since childhood are still carrying the words with them from that time, unable or unwilling to give them up. Verbal abuse replays in later years as the buried memories reappear along with the same abusive words from critical parent, teachers and peers. We hang on to abusive words and situations longer when they come from people who should have loved us but didn't. In later life those who had their self-confidence diminished as children, will often connect to verbally abusive partners whose words relate to words that have already become a familiar pattern.

A constant buildup of wax in the ears, which occurs again after removal, indicates an attachment to the words that hurt us so deeply. Words to be used against parents who we blame for our failures, used as a weapon for whatever our needs and

The Body's Emotional Imprint

wants are, making them pay the price—often monetary—for our unhappy childhood. What words did we hear as a child that we are still unwilling to release so that we can move on with our lives?

When the elderly have hearing problems and refuse to go to a doctor, it's usually out of fear of having to wear a hearing aid. In many cases it may just be a wax buildup, but the fear of being told by a doctor that their hearing is failing, stops them from seeking help—leaving those around them to believe it really is a hearing loss. The constant pressure from the family to check out their hearing may be one of the causes for the wax buildup, while another may be the words the family is saying about moving them into a nursing home.

In the past, adults hit their children much more than they do today, and the ears were often on the receiving end. The idea was to force the child to listen, but hitting the ears probably damaged their hearing so that they really couldn't hear well—causing some of them to be labeled slow learners. Today, very loud music affects the hearing of the young, especially those wearing headphones, in the same way, as it damages the ear drums. But who or what are they trying to block out? Is it an act of distancing themselves from others, or a desire to live in their own, safe world while the one outside becomes more dangerous?

Hearing is also about balance and balance can be connected to walking and moving forward, and to how balanced our lives are between work and play. Do we have balance in our work and home life, or is it all out of balance?

When we listen, especially to lectures, we often turn our head a little so that one ear is able to hear a little more than the other. Is the lecture about a left- or right-brain topic, and which side are we tuning in to? Are we hearing something new and interesting, or an opinion we are opposed to, making us listen a little harder as their opinion doesn't mirror our own?

Hearing isn't always the problem though, as the impairment may just be a flaking or constant itching of the skin around the ears that has erupted from words that we are trying to scratch out, an irritation that needs to be dealt with or a problem we don't wish to hear about. But whose words are we trying to remove? A family member who is asking us for a favor? A verbally abusive boss? A mother-in-law who always has something negative to say about our parenting skills?

When dealing with hearing loss it's also important to note that many pharmaceutical drugs, known collectively as ototoxic (having a toxic effect on the ears), including antibiotics, can affect balance, cause tinnitus, and temporary or permanent damage. As many of these drugs are given to the elderly we may think their hearing loss is related to the aging process, when in reality, it's drug-related. The effects of drugs taken on a regular basis can be accumulative and may not show up as a hearing loss until weeks or months after they are first taken, so it's important to find out which drugs will be administered, especially if there is already a hearing loss.

Words

The ears are related to balance—an even distribution of opinions and ideas—and balance is connected to the inner ear. Lack of balance is attached to words coming in that we may disagree with or words that we are unable to digest as we say "I'm not hearing him" or "I'm not on his wavelength."

When we can't process information, it's generally because it's coming in too fast or because we already have too much information. Or we are hearing too many negative words and need to hear more positive ones to bring our hearing back into balance.

"I'll smack his ears" was often said by parents who hit their children to make them behave, but taking away hearing ability leaves the one speaking the words with the power and the hard-of-hearing powerless. We tend to do the same thing to the elderly when we talk as if they can't hear.

We "turn a deaf ear" to those we don't want to listen to, or our words "fall on deaf ears" as we make the excuse that "he refused to hear my argument." In truth we may not be presenting the argument very well. We tend to close out people we have little respect for, but the problem may be that we prefer not to listen to their side of the story because their opinion doesn't mirror our own. Hearing and speaking are linked to clarity, and if our thoughts are muddled, our listening and speaking skills also becomes difficult. Speaking requires that we are able to put one word after the other to form a coherent sentence for others to understand. An out-of-balance nervous system can scramble speech when someone has taken too many drugs as it slows the brain's ability to receive and transmit messages.

Rush Limbaugh, known as the "big mouth" of talk radio, acknowledged in 2001 that he was almost completely deaf. In 2003 he admitted being addicted to prescription pain medications such as oxycodone, which is known to cause deafness.

Hearing well is connected to good health and being satisfied with the world in general, and those we consider to be "good listeners" are generally people who care about others or find listening to others enriching, especially if they are hearing something new. When the hearing starts to go, often later in life, it's usually caused by hearing things that reflect aging and feeling unwanted. Very often we are unaware of how important and hurtful our words can be to those around us and pronounce that "they can't hear us," when in fact they are really "selecting" what they wish to hear.

People who don't talk much generally listen well, while those who talk constantly may keep talking out of fear of rejection as they stop the words of others from coming in, words that may be hurtful. To "give him an earful" is to vent or put people in their place and can come from feeling powerless in a situation. Venting doesn't require an action.

Many times, we tune out the very people we are supposed to listen to, such as parents and those in authority. "I didn't listen to my doctor" can mean that either the communication between patient and doctor is poor, or the patient doesn't respect the doctor enough to listen, indicating a need to change to a doctor who's words will be worth listening to. Not listening can also indicate that the doctor is saying something negative, perhaps that surgery is needed, or a different prescription, or that the patient should move into an assisted living home, or go on a diet.

Parents who don't listen to their children and are not willing to give the child the respect they deserve, complain that the information is "going in one ear and out the other" implying that there is nothing between the ears to hold in the information. When this happens, the child will often respond by "tuning them out" so that neither side is listening.

This same scenario, of course, can be played out with a spouse, coworker or business partner, but are we the one not hearing the words, or is the other person not wanting to hear us? Maybe both parties need to open up communication to bring "music to the ears" and bring harmony into the space— and a balanced perspective.

The opposite of closing down our hearing is to "prick up our ears," which we do when something is said that we feel is interesting and worth hearing. Animals do the same thing when listening to slight sounds. When we "pin back the ears" on someone else, however, it is usually to reprimand them so that they will listen to us. It's the opposite of what we do when we want to hear ourselves speak, or hear something very carefully. Then we cup our hands over our ears or curve the ears forwards, "bending an ear," in order to hear clearly, although, bending the ears of others forces them to listen to us.

When we are "up to our ears" in something, then we are deeply involved in a situation that is detrimental. The ears are close to the top of the head and if we have "had our fill" then the problem may be beyond solving, especially if it is related to money, or someone's addictive behavior that is destroying a relationship. Up to our ears implies that we can no longer see or hear anything, so we may have reached our limit or have no solution to a problem. At this point we may need to seek help from others who are able to hear another side to things—and a solution.

Words that make us feel wanted and happy don't "hurt the ears." Unfortunately, as more and more of us move into cities, so more technology is available to block out the noise of machines, vehicles and people. But closing down our hearing also closes out the sounds of nature: birds singing, the wind whistling, the ocean roaring, and that is probably why we are able to destroy nature so easily? Perhaps if we removed the earphones and took more trips out of the city to heal our hearing, then we could improve our ability to communicate with others who don't necessarily speak our language.

See Nose, Mouth for additional information.

The Body's Emotional Imprint

EYES – Allergies

Basic Anatomy

The eyes are the visual apparatus for seeing and consist of two equal and slightly asymmetrical spheres. Most eyes are about 1 inch in diameter and fit into the eye socket, called the orbital cavity. The eye is a complex system comprised of many layers, starting with the cornea at the front and ending with the optic nerve at the back.

The cornea is a lens that curves over the front surface of the iris and pupil and is transparent in order to allow light into the back of the eye. The white part of the eye, called the sclera, protects the inner eye, while the blood vessels which are visible on the surface, nourish the sclera with oxygen and nutrients. Between the cornea and the iris is a space called the anterior chamber, which is filled with fluid to help nourish the cornea and lens.

The iris is the pigmented part of the eye which has a small opening in the center called the pupil. The amount of light coming into the eye is controlled by the pupil as it opens and closes like a camera shutter, while eye color is created by the type of pigment in the iris, which is determined by inherited genes from parents. There are three true colors in the iris: blue, brown and amber. Brown is the most common color and green the least. Other shades vary according to the amount of melanin pigment distributed within the iris, which also protects the eyes from the sun.

The cornea works together with the lens, a clear, flexible structure located behind the iris, to help focus light onto the retina. Behind the lens and in front of the retina is the vitreous cavity, which fills 2/3 of the eye with a gel-like fluid called the vitreous humor, and helps maintain the shape of the eye.

The retina acts like film in a camera to create an image. As light strikes the retina, a chemical reaction occurs sending electrical signals through the nerve cells into the optic nerve and into the brain, which then converts the information into images. Millions of tiny nerve fibers converge to form the optic nerve. The retina sees images upside down, but the brain turns them right side up so that we can interpret them as the image we think we see initially.

Eye movement is controlled by six muscles attached at the sides, top and base of the eye that allow it to move left, right, up, down and diagonally.

Emotional disharmony

Eyes and ears are closely linked and being more or less the same level on the head, are both involved in processing information. We make eye contact with people as an act of respect, or to stand our ground against someone intimidating. We stare into space when what we envision is better than the real image in front of us. We close our eyes and nod off when we are bored, indicating that we don't feel the need to stay awake. But if eyes are the windows on the world, then why do so many of us have eyesight problems?

Eyes are for looking both near and far, and normal vision can easily alternate between the two without a problem, but when the eyes don't focus well, then eyeglasses or contact lenses compensate for the discrepancies. Whether we are near sighted—able to see objects nearby but not those at a distance—or far sighted, which is the reverse, depends on which we see more clearly, the present or the future. Astigmatism is caused by a distortion of the cornea sphere and usually occurs because we have a distorted view of our surroundings and relationships. When eyeballs protrude, however, it usually signifies a problem with the thyroid.

As we age, our eyesight changes and our near sight becomes less clear, while distance often becomes clearer. The implication is that we don't want to see what's before us as it involves aging, so it's much better to see a future that we may never get to. Blurred vision suggests a life that is slowly going out of focus, perhaps from lack of stimulating company, or a blurring between middle age and old age and the expectations of others. Often we are told that certain behavior and dress is unacceptable as we get older, forcing us to withdraw from life instead of living the type of life we want. The quality of our eyesight, though, relates less to aging than to what we want to see and to the health of the muscles that encircle and attach to the eyes.

The intricate weaving of neck muscles which connect from the shoulder up to the back of the ear and from the clavicle shoulder bone to the jaw and eye sockets, can cause tension and have a significant effect on our eyesight as we tend to hold stress in the upper back and shoulder area. Children today are wearing glasses at a much younger age than earlier, but how much of it is from the stress being placed on them in situations they are incapable of handling: a heavy load of school work, getting good grades, being pushed into things they don't feel ready for, feeling peer pressure to join a group, and being pushed into sports and other outside activities that they'd rather not participate in?

During the aging process the eyes seems to shrink back into the eye sockets. In reality, it is the reduction of fat around the eye socket that makes the eyeball seem smaller. The eyeball, for some, seems to retreat from view, just as many elderly feel the need to retreat from an uncaring society and the effects of aging. Cataracts cover the eyes with a very thin film, which makes it difficult to see clearly, and many elderly have cataracts in later years, finding it more and more difficult to bring things into focus: family members who don't visit often, money worries, visits to the doctor's office, seeing their friends die. They experience a blurring of reality as the fear of getting old increases and their energy contracts and distorts what the eye sees and how it sees.

Allergies often cause the eyes to tear, which feels like the need to cry. Sneezing is an irritation that we want to sneeze out and away from us violently. Usually the sneezing takes place when we enter a new environment such as a car, train, or plane that is taking us to a destination that we don't wish to go to: a workplace, a meeting, a wedding that we'd rather not attend. An irritating situation that has gone up into the nose or into the eyes and is causing an annoyance.

We presume allergic reactions comes from dust or pollen, or from bad air quality, but they also come from situations that are not good for us, or people who will cause us problems. Does the sneezing or allergic reaction happen with the same people around, in the same place? Are we working in a sick environment? Or are we really feeling sad about a past situation that was never resolved, an anger at the way things turned out, or a parting of ways? Going back to when the allergic reaction first happened will often show us what the irritant was that started it—person or situation. Where were we living? Who were we with? We presume that once we have

The Body's Emotional Imprint

allergies we always will, but allergies come and go depending on what our connection is to the thing that caused the reaction.

Eyes that constantly water are really tears not shed, an inability to grieve at the time of someone's death, or the end of a situation that was never fully addressed. Dry eyes, on the other hand, can reflect a desire not to show emotions for something in the past that we refuse to acknowledge, and as we hold the hurt inside and refuse to cry, the eyes dry out. If it affects only one eye, then we need to understand who may have been responsible for the unshed tears or the reason for an unresolved conflict—a bitter divorce, the death of an abusive parent, or the need to be strong after a spouse has died. If both eyes are affected then it can indicate something external, such as as being fired from a job or losing a home.

Conjunctivitis, also known as pink eye, is a virus, bacteria or allergic reaction, and is a more debilitating and serious eye infection which can take a few days to clear. A severe case will be affected by any kind of light, even daylight, making it impossible to go out without dark glasses. What are we trying to block out and why are we trying to stay in the dark? Or are we being kept in the dark about a situation? What is happening in our life that we no longer want to see or acknowledge?

Children sometimes experience crossed eyes, but this suggests the wiring of the brain was crossed by conflicting emotions, probably before birth. Many things are passed through the mother even before the baby is born, especially emotional and physical upsets, so it's important to go back to how the mother was feeling before the birth. If the crossed eyes happen when the child is a little older, then the wiring has crossed because of something emotional that they are unable to make sense of. Words from parents may be conflicting, leading the child to receive crossed messages from both the mother and the father with one saying one thing, the other something different.

Most of us have one eye that has better vision than the other, is a different shape or more open or closed. All these things represent how far we can see, what we can see, if we want to see, and which side we favor to see. An eye that is damaged or has to be removed can relate to the future and if it holds anything we really want to see. Or we may feel that we cannot see ourselves represented in the future.

It's interesting to compare the type size in books today with those in antique books. The type size in newer books has grown as has the space between the lines. This is partly to fill books and make them look bigger than they really are, but it may also be because we no longer have the time to read entire books and bigger type makes it easier to scan pages.

Words
Many people say, "I just can't see it." in response to being asked to see something someone else's way. Having to deal with a vision that is not our own, we may "stare them down" in the hope that they will back down and see our stronger vision. But if we ask others to "clarify" the situation, then maybe a solution could be found "right in front of our eyes." Often simple answers are the most difficult to see.

"I don't see how we're going to do it " or "I must be blind" all indicate a tiredness due to constantly having to come up with solutions; perhaps for family or coworkers who don't pull their weight, or an elderly parent who can no longer make decisions for themselves. It also indicates a much deeper health problem than the eyes, perhaps an adrenal or thyroid problem that needs attention.

When we are in good health, we talk of "eyes that sparkle," which they do when we are in love and well cared for. We use positive words for how well we can see things in the future, such as "I see it so clearly" and we "see eye to eye" with others. If we are "blinded by the light," which animals often are as they are caught like "deer in the headlights," we may not see a situation clearly, or are being mislead by someone and are so blind to what's going on that we make a wrong decision.

Singer Ray Charles wasn't born blind but started to lose his eyesight at the age of five years -- shortly after witnessing the drowning death of his younger brother. By the age of 7 he was totally blind.

On the other hand, light is bright and it could be the opening up to new experiences and to finally "seeing the light." Needing light to see any situation entails shining the light from somewhere else, and often the light comes from the opinions of others if we are willing to listen closely to what they have to say. Stubbornness can lead to bad decisions if we refuse to "give in" to someone else.

Wanting to be "very clear about my next move" can refer to an actual move to another home, city, country, or a career move. It reflects a desire to finally get it right, a need to move on, either from people or a job that is no longer working. Asking others to be "clear about their next move" often indicates that the one saying the words to another is fed up with things not working out and wants the next move, figuratively or physical, to be the right one. It could be someone speaking about a relationship or a boss talking to the workers, but it implies that patience is running thin. Getting "clear" about any situation means being able to see the entire picture from all directions.

Laughter and tears are closely connected, which is why many parents tell kids who laugh too much that there will be "tears before bedtime." Tears flow through the eyes and are linked to emotional highs and lows. We cry for those departed, those being born and everything in between, with tears of joy and tears of sadness. Tears well up when we are touched by some event, and we are "moved to tears" with music that can "bring tears to our eyes." We cry when we are breaking up, losing a job, angry, hurt or remorseful. Tears represent strong emotions that we feel a need to express, which is why women will often say, " I feel so much better after a good cry." Tears are a release of all the pent-up emotions which then allow clarity to return.

If we choose wrong words, the way we speak around children will sometimes limit their efforts. If we tell them that they are not "putting enough effort into it" we presume they are being lazy, when in fact, they may not be able to do what has been asked. In an educational situation kids will say of their teacher, "I just couldn't see what he was talking about" as they "fumble around in the dark" looking for solutions. They may be out of their depth with the curriculum and don't know what to do next, so it's worth listening to kids to hear what they are really having problems with. Is it the subject or the teacher? Are they really unable to do the work or just have a different interpretation on how it should be done? The educational system accommodates only one way of learning when there are many ways—some students are visual, some are audial, some need a hands-on approach.

Someone who has "fixed his eyes on the prize" is not easily derailed and defeated, unlike people who have "limited vision." In a work situation it's important to be surrounded by "can do" people who do see down the road, especially if it's our own business. When we go into a situation with our "eyes wide open" we have taken into account all eventualities and we take full responsibility for our actions. Eyes that are wide open see the future clearly, ready to "make eye contact" with everyone we meet.

Perfect eyesight signifies a balanced outlook and an ability to "see both sides" of a situation, so maybe we should choose politicians by how good their eyesight is!

See Nose, Thyroid, Adrenals, Right/Left side for additional information.

FEET – Toes

Basic Anatomy

One quarter of all the bones in the human body are in the feet, with 26 bones in each foot, 14 of which form the toes. Ligaments, which connect one bone to another and give strength to joints, are composed of tough, fibrous, dense strands of collagen. They hold the joint in place and give support to the inside and outside of the foot, while tendons, which connect muscles to bones, allow the foot flexibility as it lifts and bends. The largest and strongest tendon in the body is the Achilles tendon, which connects the heel to the calf muscle—the area runners often damage.

In a healthy foot the toes should be straight and the foot well formed, strong and flexible. Toes, which do the same grasping action as the fingers, help to stabilize the foot when walking. The foot is divided into three areas: the hindfoot, midfoot and forefoot. The bones of the toes are called phalanges and the forefoot consists of the big toe, with two bones, and four smaller toes, made up of three jointed bones each. The phalanges are connected to bones called metatarsals, elongated bones that form the ball of the foot. This area bears the weight of the body as it thrusts forward during walking and running, and also provides balance.

The midfoot provides shock absorbers in the form of five tarsal bones and connects the mid section to the forefoot at one end and the hindfoot on the other by way of muscles and the plantar fascia—the arch ligament. The plantar fascia is thick connective tissue beneath the foot which supports the arch and runs from the heelbone to the metatarsal bones.

The Body's Emotional Imprint

The hindfoot links the midfoot to the ankle by way of the talus—the bone that connects to the two bones of the lower leg to form the ankle—and the calcaneus, or heelbone, which is the largest bone in the foot and forms the base of the heel, and is cushioned by a layer of fat.

Muscles, tendons and ligaments which stabilize and allow movement, run along the surfaces of the foot to form a base for running, jumping and standing on the toes.

Emotional disharmony

Physical problems often start with the feet, but they are usually the last thing we take care of. We pay attention to the body first, and the feet only when we have difficulty walking. Feet keep us standing firmly in place, and when we walk and place one foot in front of the other, they support us as we move towards places and the things that we want. They are about intention, a plan and a will to take us where we want to go.

Sometimes only one foot wants to move while the other hesitates, reflecting how we feel about our masculine and feminine side, so if the two sides are in conflict, the end result will be a trip or a fall. Do we feeling vulnerable, unsure of our strength in dealing with a situation?—reflecting the left side. Or do we feel strong enough to step forward and ask for what we want?—the the right side.

If we are out of balance, then the soles of our footwear will indicate where the imbalance is by the area that has worn down. Heels that are worn down shows a strong intent, but can also signify someone who is pushing too hard. Worn at the ball of the foot show lack of ability to move as high as we'd like, or a feeling of imbalance. If worn at the inner sides, then we internalize things and keep to ourselves.

Feet, quite literally, keep us grounded, so how grounded do we feel? If we don't feel that the ground can support us then we trip, and tripping over things indicated we are not sure-footed enough in our lives to walk directly to what we want. Sometimes we can catch ourselves before falling, while at other times we take a tumble. How much of the body hits the ground represents how insecure we feel. A hand may save us by grabbing onto something before we fall, and at other times we may hit our face on the ground with the rest of the body following. But are we moving to a place we want, or a place we are fearful of going to? Are we going to see some-one we want to meet, or someone to whom we feel inferior?

Children and older people often trip as they are not sure of the ground below them. For the elderly it reflects how sup-ported they feel as they age, and for children it is about not understanding their connection to the world around them, or their place in it, or in some cases, where they fit in.

Walking with feet turned inwards—called pigeon-toed— shows a desire to turn inwards on ourselves and not out-wards towards others. But walking with feet turned inwards doesn't support us as easily as if we placed our feet straight and firmly on the ground. Today may young people walk pigeon-toed, sometimes because of being overweight, and at other times because the knee has turned inwards and forced the ankle to twist too. Usually this stance wears down the inside part of the sole, which is the same as wearing down our inner soul. We have a feeling of being detached from society and of not fitting in. It can also be that we prefer not to intrude into the space of others, or we lack the confidence to take up the space we need.

Bunions, a bump on the inner side of the foot at the base of the big toe, is concentrated energy that distorts the toe, which then pushes against all the other toes causing them, too, to fall out of alignment. A bunion produces pain and walking difficulty, but is also a distortion of our interpretation of the world in general, just as our congealed thoughts have formed the bunion. We blame the deformity on badly fitting shoes, but a healthy foot will overcome shoes that are too tight, just as we humans can overcome difficulties. Forcing the foot into a shoe that is too tight, though, comes from vanity and a wanting to be a Cinderella whose slipper fits perfectly so that the handsome prince will emerge to sweep us off our feet. It reflects the need to have others take care of us, which the big toe does to the smaller toes as it stabilizes the foot. Bunions are the message that the prince hasn't arrived and we won't be leading a fairy tale existence, and to accept that reality.

Swollen feet are usually caused by an excess of fluid in the muscles and can be painful to walk on, but if the fluid is not released, then emotions that caused the fluid buildup are also not released. Fluid, which should flow easily, represents unshed tears, and in the feet is related to being stuck and making wrong decisions, such as living or moving to the wrong place. We may be living in a place or with a situation that we dislike, but saying so may then force us to move on again, a move that could be painful. So the emotions stay bottled up, just as the fluid stays bottled up and just as we stay bottled up in the same place, same job, same relationship, with the same problems. Or, we are hanging on to a problem that refuses to flow out.

Flat feet plod with no spring to the walk, no flexibility, no shape to life, no definition. We have no ability to express our needs or expectations. A high instep, however, is the opposite as it shows high expectations, but if the foot is injured, those expectations can be dashed, which often happens to athletes and dancers. We may start off with healthy feet and high insteps, only to find later in life, that the instep has flattened out just as our lives have leveled out. We may also have an elevated sense of ourselves that doesn't represent reality.

When we walk, the heel usually meets the ground first, and if we look at our own shoes and those of others, the heel is often where the shoe wears away first as the heel connects to the ground too forcefully. We place the heel down too firmly when we are trying to get, and stay, grounded. We are trying to connect, trying to hold on, trying desperately to move ahead to where we want to be, in business or in life.

Humans have five toes on each foot, although we can walk with fewer if we have to, and they give us balance and stability by giving us the ability to cling to things. Gnarled and twisted toes reveal compressed energy and produces an inability to cling, either to life, a situation or a person. We may feel needy and unsure of our future path but are too weak to wrap our toes onto the pathway that would take us to a better place. Toes that curl under are trying to cling to an unsafe surface and lack the courage to take the plunge to a safer environment, and in doing so, limit our intent. Are we clinging to outworn ideas we have outgrown? Or memories we should have released? Toenails protect the ends of the toes, but an ingrown nail turns back on itself from fear of not being protected and taken care of if we venture out.

The Body's Emotional Imprint

Overlapping toes are crowded and fighting for space, fighting to be heard in a crowded world, an energy twisted by twisted thoughts. The big toe indicates a large problem, the small toe something much smaller, although all toes need their own space to grow into healthy units. What are we crowding together that we won't allow space between? Ourselves, or others? We can do damage to ourselves by trying to keep others down, sometimes by the guilt of an action and at other times by our self-loathing at not being able to control the hostility and anger we feel. Crowding others out may also be related to not wanting to share space, love, possessions, or money, with siblings or others we view as a threat.

When we feel "really grounded" we often use our clench fist sideways to denote the action of being grounded, as if we are pounding stakes into the ground. But it can also have negative connotations if it refers to a person we really want to pound into the ground.

Feet can also be defiant as they stamp and stomp and can be very militaristic when collectively they march in unison as an army; a stomping action that can instill fear in others who have not joined the group. Showing solidarity is all about "being in step" with others. We can dance in a group, too, which also brings community together, not with intimidation but as joy, so the pressure of the foot on the ground can be pleasurable or a means of force.

Words

We have many sayings for feet, probably because of its use in moving and keeping us on the the ground, but if we don't feel secure, then we talk of "not feeling grounded" as if it won't support us. When we don't feel grounded we talk of feeling "spacey" and "lightheaded" and not able to attend to the things that need our attention. Something is happening in our heads that will not allow the thoughts to pass further down so that we can take action with the feet.

When the feet are "planted firmly on the ground," we feel in complete control of a situation and relate well to everyone and everything. We have a total consciousness that can't be derailed. Anything to do with the ground is about stability as we stand on a rock base—the planet—but if we imagine that the rock is crumbling then our stability will crumble too, and it's interesting that today, as we destroy the planet with drilling, blasting and mountain topping, we are all feeling less grounded and secure. We may no longer be "sure-footed" about our progress in life or that we will have a life, but if we can "find our feet again," then we will overcome obstacle in our path and navigate around them.

> There are 52 bones in the feet, a quarter of all the bones in the human body.

Lack of stability can come from an insecure childhood, constantly moving from place to place, or from emotional insecurity, with parents who argued or threatened divorce, or some other family upheaval such as a death. Children are expected to "bounce back" after a traumatic event, but most of the time we carry the event with us, to reappear later in life as insecurity that leads us into a bad relationship, marriage or an overbearing partnership.

The words we use to describe how we feel about our feet have either a negative or positive connotation, with not much in between, which implies that we are either having problems walking or we don't have to think about the action. We can "dance the night away" or "drag our feet." And are either "swept off our feet" or "tripping over our own feet." If we feel good about life then we use the word "dance" to indicate how light hearted we feel. We are floating through life as if our feet "never touched the ground." Or we "quicken the pace" to get to a pleasant destination much faster.

On the other hand if we "step on someone's toes" and "tap dance around the situation" we are clumsy and prefer not to deal with an issue, or have dealt with it in a graceless manner; perhaps involving money, work or a social scene. We ask others to "step out of your comfort zone" when we want them to take a chance and expand their horizon. On the other hand, we may be asking them to take a chance on our behalf, while they are not ready to take the step. So are we really the one who needs encouragement, or are they? Are we really asking for their need, or our own?

Walking is an unconscious action that only becomes a conscious undertaking when it is an effort to place one foot in front of the other. At that point it becomes difficult to be motivated enough to give impetus to the action, whether it's physical or emotional. Not walking well can come from being stuck in a low-paying job, losing a job, or just losing confidence. Something that "slips away" from us, just as we slip physically from lack of attention and weakened muscles, leaving us "unsure of our footing."

A corn, which is extremely painful, is a thickening of the skin formed in response to excess pressure being placed on it. Corns usually affect the toes and often return if not dealt with. A "sore point" on the toe indicates some problem that has not been resolved or is taking a great deal of effort and time. Sore points often happen in families when no one can agree on a course of action, or at work when a coworker creates a painful situation for the other workers. But who is suffering from the corn, the person creating the disturbing situation or those who are on the receiving end? So "bite the bullet" and relieve the pressure by taking action on the problem; otherwise it will keep recurring.

Women are often too timid to put their "best foot forward" and instead they step back while allowing others to step forwards, causing resentment that turns inwards and a foot problem that will slow any future advancement. Many people say " I don't feel I'm getting anywhere" to describe their lack of progress or upward mobility in a job, or even in finding a job, as they "tread water." We may want to "stand on our own two feet," but being "stuck in one place" won't move us to a better place, especially if we "dig our heels in" and refuse help.

We tend to "cling to life" when all hope has gone, but maybe the clinging is the problem, especially when we should "walk away" from a marriage that has finished. Or perhaps we are too fearful to "walk away." The state of the feet gives an indication on how high our intentions are and whether or not we are capable of getting there.

See Ankle, Knees and Hands for additional information

GALL BLADDER

Basic Anatomy

The gall bladder is a small storage sac, three to four inches long, that sits just under the liver. Its function is to collect bile from the liver and store it until needed for the digestive process and then pass it along to the duodenum—the hollow jointed tube about 10" -12" long which is the first part of the small intestine.

Bile is a thick yellow-green substance containing water, mineral salts, cholesterol, fats, bile acids, phospholipids and bilirubin, and assists in the process of breaking down fats to make them water soluble. It gets its color from a pigment called bilirubin, derived from decomposed red blood cells which are part of the process that turns feces brown. Without bile activity, the feces will be grayish white in color and streaked with undigested fat. Toxins from the liver—bacteria, viruses, drugs and other foreign substances—are also removed via bile.

Gallstones are hard masses that collect in the bile duct and block the flow into the duodenum. They are usually composed of cholesterol, calcium carbonate and bilirubin. Eighty per cent of bile is reused during a meal, with the remaining 20% eliminated in the feces along with the excess of cholesterol, which, if not excreted, can form into a gallstone.

Emotional disharmony

Bile it bitter, so the emotional connection to this area is about bitterness and resentment. It could be resentment at a past event or something much closer. Bitterness is a bad taste in the mouth. We spit out anything tasting very bitter as it spoils the taste of other things: things that could, if we let them, taste good and satisfying. So what could we be savoring in life, but are too angry and resentful to try? Is someone making us bitter? And what, or who, are we resentful of: a family member, coworker, or a situation we feel that we are stuck with? A business relationship we signed up for? Or a situation we knew was bad from the start but entered into anyway? Or a relationship that has gone sour? Are we feeling unappreciated? Passed over for a job? Or has life passed us by? And what are we hoping to block in others—movement, happiness, sweetness—but are really obstructing in ourselves.

The gall bladder is a collection station, storing the bile before moving it along, but here we also hang onto emotions by not allowing them to move on to the digestive system, where foods/emotions are broken down. Allowing bile to bottle up at this point is also about bottling up the sourness instead of letting it flow on and out. But are we the one who is being cruel, or is someone directing their nastiness at us, and what words would we like to spit at others in return—a partner, coworker, parent, siblings?

Gallstones can be as small as a grain of sand or as large as a golf ball, and can develop into just one large stone or hundreds of tiny ones. How big the stone is, will indicates the size of the resentment and whether it is aimed a just one person or at many. Are we blaming others for our own bad judgment or lack of initiative, or did they actually do something behind our backs? Or, have we grown the problem out of all proportion?

Stones are hard to break down and difficult to move, but smaller stones can be picked up and thrown, so who or what would be the target if we could throw them? Allowing the resentment to build into something that is difficult to move may block our own exit, but where are we trying to move to? Another job, a new location, marriage? Is someone else blocking our way or are we too afraid to stand up for what we want?

Gallstones are often prevalent in obese people, especially women over the age of forty. But obesity is a way of not letting people get close, physically or emotionally, putting up a barrier, just as the gallstone has by adding extra weight to those who are already carrying around fat deposits and not allowing the bile to break them down. Obesity shows a resistance to change and all it may bring, a resistance against being noticed.

Words

Many say, "I'm so bitter about what she/he's done to this family" when things don't work out because of someone who is standing in the way of a desired and expected outcome. "He's a bitter person" we say about others, and often the words "bitter" and "resentful" are used in the same sentence to emphasize just how far down the bitterness goes and how long it has been hanging around.

Sour people are usually "sharp tongued" and impatient, wanting to get an issue over with as fast as possible, wishing the situation to pass quickly and not linger. Unfortunately, situations that are not dealt with tend to linger, just as gallstones do, causing sharp painful attacks along with sour emotions. An over-acidic body can produce gallstones, and is an indication that we are out of balance in our lives. Acid is corrosive, which is how we feel when we talk of having an "acid tongue."

The sharpness has built up to corrode our relationships at home or at work.

If we find ourselves saying "I feel so bitter" about a situations that hasn't worked out, then we need to find the cause before it can eat its way through the relationship that caused the ill will. Who stopped it from working out, others or ourselves? Are we the one who is making it into a bitter experience? Very often we sabotage ourselves when we feel insecure about moving to a new job or taking on more responsibility, and we do and say things we wouldn't normally, which give the wrong impression to the people we are trying to impress. Then when things don't work out, resentment builds and we blame others as we are forced to "swallow defeat," telling everyone that "it's a bitter pill to swallow." However, after we swallow it we then just let it sit there and stagnate into a grudge rather than allowing it to run a natural course.

John Ashcroft, controversial U.S. Attorney General from 2001-2005, initiated the creation of Operation TIPS, in which workers and government employees would inform on any suspicious behavior of others while performing their duties. In 2004, Ashcroft was diagnosed with a severe case of Gallstone Pancreatitis and had to have his gallbladder removed.

The word "gall" is used to indicate that someone has had the temerity to do something against us. "The gall of it!" we spit out. But lack of gall on our part often indicates timidity and indecision, allowing other to push us aside—often in a work situation where others are promoted over us, or resentment may arise at home when the family expects us to do all the work.

The Body's Emotional Imprint

The dictionary defines "gall" as a "chronic irritation,"—something that frets and wears away by friction. What situation have we allowed to grind us down? Is it affecting our health in other areas too? Is a marriage eroding our confidence; the responsibility of taking care of aging parents exhausting us, too many long hours at work? Or are people trying to make us change our minds on a subject?

The word "bile" suggests something unpleasant and as we spit the word out, we can smell the offensive odor that bile gives off. We can see the horrible color, like a stagnating pond where nothing is moving, just like an unpleasant situation that we need to move away from, a situation that is forcing us to become ill-natured. A situation that is forcing us to stagnate when what we really want is something new and exciting.

Perhaps the words that we really want to say, we are not able to say. But if we could say those words instead of internalizing them, who would we say them to? The area where bile rests is in the chest, and often we say "I need to get it off my chest" to indicate that the emotions are just sitting there, crushing the air out of us.

See Liver and Chest for additional information.

GENITALS

Basic Anatomy

The male reproductive system is also part of the urinary system and consists of the penis, scrotum, testicles, vas deferens, seminal vesicles, prostate gland and the urethra. The penis is cylindrical in shape and contains the urethra, which opens externally at the tip of the penis to allow urine to be expelled from the body and semen to be delivered into the vagina during sexual intercourse, which it does by filling with blood to give it an erect form when aroused.

The vas deferens is a tube attached to the testicles that transport sperm cells, after they develop in the testes, into the seminal vesicles. Located behind the prostate, the seminal vesicle, along with the prostate, produce a fluid that mixes with the sperm to produce semen. During ejaculation the muscles surrounding the area contract and push out the sperm and fluid through the urethra.

The scrotum, a thin sac of skin and muscle that hangs below the penis, contain the testes. There are two testicles, usually about 1.5 – 2 inches long and an inch in diameter, that are responsible for sperm and testosterone—the male sex hormone. The scrotum allows the testicles to hang slightly away from the body to keeps them a little cooler than the rest of the body, which is needed for optimal sperm development. There is evidence today to suggest that in industrialized nations the testes' size and weight have been progressively shrinking and sperm count decreasing, which suggest that environment, lifestyle and chemicals are disrupting development.

Male circumcision is the removal of the foreskin from the penis. Many believe that the foreskin should be removed for cleanliness or religious reasons, although today there is little medical evidence to support the former idea, and fewer couples willing to accept it for their sons.

The female reproductive system is located entirely in the pelvis and is divided into the inner and outer genital organs. The outer ones are the major and minor labia and the clitoris, the inner organs consist of the ovaries, fallopian tubes, uterus and vagina. Covering the opening of the vagina is the vulva, which is the name for the collective outer genitalia. The major labia are a pair of thick folds of fatty tissue which surround the minor labia, thinner folds of skin that enclose the vaginal opening. The clitoris, which contains many nerve endings that serve as a sensory organ for sexual pleasure, is also enclosed within the labia.

The vagina is an elastic, muscular tube about 3 to 5 inches long protected by mucous membranes. It connects the uterus to the exterior of the body and serves as the receptacle for the penis during sexual intercourse and the birth canal in childbirth, and provides a route for menstrual blood to exit the body from the uterus. Girls are born with hundreds of thousands of eggs in the ovaries, which remain inactive until puberty when the pituitary gland starts to make hormones that stimulate the ovaries. If the eggs are not fertilized by sperm, then they leave the body with blood and tissue from the inner lining of the uterus—the process called menstruation. Once the cycle stops, usually around the age of 50, menopause begins.

Emotional disharmony

Our genital area is connected to trust, both of ourselves and others, and how we feel about nakedness, sexuality and the sexual act. We may wear skimpy bikinis, even go topless, but we keep the genital area covered to keep secret something of value that we can withhold or share—or even sell.

The level of comfort we feel in showing our genitals to others relates to how well the family handled its own sexuality. If we grew up detecting embarrassment and humiliation to anything regarding nudity and sexuality, then we usually fall on one of two side, becoming either uptight about all things sexual in nature, or promiscuous in order to be defiant. Having a balanced outlook on reproduction and nudity will lead to emotional balance in relationships. Religion has also had a strong influence on society's sexual mores and a profound effect on how we view our own bodies and those of others, and how we view nudity in general. It's difficult to discard the "good" girl image that religion has set up.

For women, nudity often equates with a high degree of emotional vulnerability, but for men, much less true, as nudity is related to the principle of power. In wars the genital area is associated with torture and rape—of both men and women—used, as in all situations concerning sexual abuse, as weapons of power and control and to keep the victim feeling powerless.

The vagina is where the man enter the woman, either for sexual intimacy, procreation, or power, and troubles here relate to how comfortable we feel with our partner and whether or not we feel violated. Vaginal infections signify a feeling of being used or not wanting to have sex but participating in the act anyway. The genitals lie in the pelvic area, where women conceive and give birth, and can show how secure we feel partnering with another man or woman in order to to bring the project—which a birth is for some women—to climax. It can also relate to partnering in a new business, a marriage, or a trip.

The penis, for men, represents virility and manhood and so any negativity around the genital area signifies lack of worth and feelings of inadequacy, a fear of not being able to perform, either sexually, at work or, in society. Retirement often produces sexual worries, and even though the initial problem is loss of status and not loss of virility, drugs are often given for the lack of libido. The inability to perform also reflects a lack of involvement in society as the opportunities dwindle, and feeling unnecessary increases. This loss, then plays out in the most vulnerable area of the body, the sexual organs. An erect penis, however, indicates being in control and able to command it to perform at will. Feeling virile, manly and in charge are all things men associate with being "real" men. Losing a job, a marriage, a business, can affect our self-image, much of which is attached to our sexuality and how we present it to the world.

Circumcision is an assault on the most private, sensitive and valuable part of a man, and for many, is the first real pain they feel. Some adults believe that a baby doesn't feel pain and that circumcision does little harm, but even if the circumcision itself is quick and the area around the cutting is anesthetized, what of the pain after the anesthetic wears off—often for a prolonged period of time afterwards? What emotional scars does circumcision cause?

Copulation is about energy, how we use it, and who we are willing to share it with, but in this society we receive conflicting messages as the media flaunts sexuality on the one hand, but gives us puritanical politics on the other. Feeling conflicted about sexuality can also come from a strictly religious home where copulation is considered for procreation only and where lack of engagement with a partner spurs a need to draw back and not enjoy the connecting of another, often from fear of the consequences.

Sexual abuse will also bring up strong emotions regarding the sexual act and can produce feelings of revulsion, not necessarily of the abuser, but for not fighting or reporting the abuse. We are also brought up to feel revulsion at what the genitals look like, especially when women feel vulnerable. For men, the insecurity comes from the size of the penis and how it "stacks up" compared to those of other men.

Any diseased part of the body denotes the area where we have bottled up the emotions, and problems with the genitals, such as herpes, AIDS and cancer, often connote a mistrust or anger at having shared ourselves with someone we didn't particularly want to share ourselves with, perhaps by being talked into the act, or by taking drugs and alcohol which weakened our resolve. But who is being punished? Do we feel abused, or have we abused the other party? Do we feel guilty for having forced ourselves on others, or did they force themselves on us? Where were the boundaries that we missed, the message we didn't pay attention to, or the lack of self-worth that pushed us down the wrong path?

How we view our own genitals is usually an indication of how well we will enjoy the sexual act with our partner. If we see them as something ugly that has to be kept in the dark, then partners will be kept at a distance, or we will become frigid.

Seeing the body as a celebration, of both ourselves and of our partner, will release a vibrant energy between couples.

Words

Feeling insecure about sexuality has forced us as a society to find other words for genitals—usually derogatory words. Men, especially, use jokey terms which take away the serious-ness of the word "penis." But this probably comes from par-ents who are timid about talking to their own children about anything sexual and so teach children from an early age to find alternative words for the genitals and excrement. Young boys delight in trying to gross each other out with jokey terms—and often big boys too! The less confident we feel about our sexuality and nudity, the less accurate the words are to describe it. Using the term "private parts" indicates that they are private and are shared with very few.

Men use the word "cunt" to talk about women in an offen-sive way, but usually think of their own organ as a weapon to be used against women as they talk of the penis as a "prick," "pecker," or "tool". Discomfort saying the word "penis" adds to the feeling that it is something "dirty" and not to be dis-cussed. So anything that's wrong with the health of the penis will also not be discussed, which means that "erectile dysfunc-tion" has now become a code word for "flaccid."

Impotence—unspoken by most men—is changed to the phrase "couldn't get it up" which implies that the penis was flaccid, weak, not working as it should be and going in the wrong direction. The phrase is used to describe men who have a weakness in their character and who "don't have the balls to get the job done." We talk of men—and some women—as having "balls," meaning that they are tough and not willing to back down in any situation. The inference is that balls are tough and that women with balls are "ballsy" and they take charge just like a man.

But when needed, a penis is supposed to be erect, as confident men stand erect. We "move up in the world" when we are doing well, and "upward mobility" suggests that we are going places, and those places are "up there." Any health problem we have in the entire genital area—physically or emotionally—links to how we view our status in a relationship—within the family, a work unit, or as a nation.

Women who are not comfortable with their own bodies will sometimes use the phrase "down there" to refer to their genital area, an area that many are afraid of and never investigate further. But "down there" is also where the Devil resides, and he lures us into naughty actions, especially connected to sex and fun, so sex and religion are closely linked, especially when we speak of women being in the missionary position, underneath the man. It can also denote feeling like the "underdog" if the male implies that.

> The words up and down filter into who we are as a society, with men in positions of power at the top, and women below in the missionary pose in copulation. The rich move up, while the rest are "down on their luck" or "down trodden."

The word "genital" is a catchword for all that is "down there," a place where sexual intercourse takes place, a place where urine streams from, a place where partners investigate. It's a catchall for things leaving and things coming in—invited or otherwise.

The words "up" and "down" are about our status and where we consider ourselves to be on the ladder. Are we going in the "right direction" or sliding down?

Stating "I'm not in a good place" implies that we are not doing well in life, but it can also suggest being in a "bad place" in a relationship and that it's time to get out. Perhaps someone is domineering and constantly "putting us down" or the place has become dangerous. Hearing others say these words suggests that they need help, which may mean extricating them from an abusive situation.

Men who are lazy are often told by other men to "get their finger out," which is a derogatory term meaning "Shape up." Again the word "up." If you are not going up at all times, then you are not worth much, which is why many men who are aging and have lost their work status, experience bouts of impotency and prostate problems.

See Pituitary, Prostate, Bladder, Breasts for additional information.

HAND – Fingers – Arthritis

Basic Anatomy

The hands and feet are very similar with regard to their structural make up, but except when we are sleeping, the hands are usually in constant motion: touching, holding, working or computing. The bones of the fingers, called phalanges, have two joints on the thumb and three on the remaining fingers and connect to the metacarpals, the bones that make up the hand. These in turn connect to the carpals at the wrist. The human hand has 27 bones, fourteen for the fingers, five for the metacarpals—one for each finger—and eight for the carpals.

Ligaments are tough bands of tissue that connect the bones together, and the collateral ligaments, which run down each side of each finger and thumb, prevent damage from occurring through sideways bending of the joints. The flexor tendons originate above the wrist, as do the muscles, and attach the bones of the fingers, and are responsible for the flexing of the hand and the bending of the fingers. The nerves, which carry the signals to brain and back to the muscles in order to move the hand and fingers, begin at the upper spine.

Arthritis is a painful inflammation of joints, and on the hand it usually affects the fingers, but arthritis is used to describe many different diseases and conditions of the joints and connective tissue. Osteoarthritis involves the breakdown of cartilage which provides a gliding surface for the joints to function smoothly and to act as a cushion between the bones of the joints. When the joints are worn or damaged, they often become painful with swelling, stiffness or inflammation. The condition usually affects the joints; knees, hips, wrists, elbows, fingers or spine, especially if there has been a previous injury or stress to that joint.

Rheumatoid arthritis, which is more common in women than men, is an autoimmune disease whereby the immune system mistakenly attacks the body's own tissue. It causes painful swelling, inflammation of the joints and stiffness, and can lead to bone erosion and deformity.

Men are more susceptible to gout, a form of arthritis which involves recurring attacks of stiffness, swelling or sudden burning pain of the joints—often a big toe, although it can occur in other areas—and is caused by elevated levels of uric acid and crystal deposits that form in the joints and surrounding tissue. It used to be called "the rich man's disease" since only the wealthy could afford alcohol, and rich, fatty, calorie-laden foods associated with the disease.

Emotional disharmony

We hold children's hands to keep them safe and close to us, and when we become older we hold the hands of those we love. Hands are for holding: things, people and creative projects. We can produce wonderful things with our hands, but we can also destroy the things we build.

In Western culture we shake hands as a welcome gesture when we meet others we are not familiar with. But even though our hand may clasp theirs, the arm is held away from the body which keeps them at arm's length. Other cultures greet one another with a slight bow, a hug, hands held together as if in prayer, or the kissing of each cheek. Hands can pull people up or push them down, so what we choose to do with them is indicative of who we are and how we view others in the world.

Hands speak volumes about us. We may help nature along by resculpting our face and body, but hands are exposed to the world just as they are: with no make-up, no plastic surgery. Some hands are hardworking, others are hands of leisure, some are gnarled and dry, others smooth and soft, but they all represent who we are, our feelings about what we present to others, what our hands have been used for, and the willingness to grasp at what we want.

Making a fist and holding the arm in the air is a symbol of defiance or victory—usually over others. Sports figures do this when they win, as do activists who go against the norms of society, and men show a clenched fist to threaten others. The balling up of the hand is the balling up of high emotions, but an outstretched hand is a sign of welcome. We show people and animals an outstretched hand to demonstrate that we carry no weapon and are not a threat.

When dry skin affects the hands and fingers, it is a drying up of our ability to connect, which usually translates into an unwillingness to be social, to shake hands, or to hold hands with others. Dry and cracked skin on the fingertips indicates a need to cover over who we really are, and just as fingerprints establish our true identify, the peeling away of the dry skin is a way to become someone else, someone we may like more, or a way of establishing a new identity in a new place. A new way of seeing ourselves and the world around us.

Cuts, burns and nicks on hands and fingers—which often happen as we cook—are caused by a lack of attention, either from being too familiar with the act or because our mind has wandered to other things. But wandered to what? Would we rather be doing something else? Doing it in a different location? Cooking for someone else? Sharing the meal with

The Body's Emotional Imprint

someone? When we cut our hand, the cut can be a substitute for resentment that has built up from doing the action, perhaps because we are the only one in the family expected to cook, and even though we may enjoy cooking, now we feel taken advantage of.

Cold hands indicate poor circulation and poor energy. The warm blood isn't flowing and there is a feeling of coldness to others, or coldness is coming back to us from those we love, or would like to love.

Nails are the energy at the end of the fingers and show the state of our health by how well they grow. Problems can show up as ridges, cracks, bending or discoloration and represent the emotional state that has caused the nails to deform. Strong nails show a strong constitution and allow us to go after our goals, while cracks and chips show our vulnerability in reaching out, either for people or situations we wish to move into. Brittle nails are the opposite of supple ones; they bend and crack when we have to accommodate others. Brittle people scold and being brittle implies that a "breaking point" may be close at hand. So how damaged are the nails?

Nails can also scrape, pick and gouge, both others and ourselves, and if it is ourselves that we have turned on, then what has pushed us to do the act? People with a compulsive disorder sometimes scrape their skin until it bleeds, producing blood, which is our life force as it keeps the organs going with oxygen. So who is forcing the air out of us? The color red also represents anger, so the scratching may be anger at another who won't leave us alone and we may be trying to scratch them out of our life. If we are not strong enough to ask for what we want, the scratching can be a plea for help.

Compulsion of any kind is based on a need to get things right. We know the behavior is destructive, but we can't stop ourselves. But who has set the drive in motion? A parent who was never satisfied with anything we did as a child? Someone in authority who constantly chastised us, a sibling who always picked on us? Usually we obsess about small things, which become bigger because of our compulsion to do something to control the small thing in the first place. We may obsess over a small sewing job by sewing the same area over and over again, until a hole appears in the fabric—then we have a reason to attack ourselves.

Many elderly people develop arthritis in their hands as they see little to reach out for. Fingers become crooked as they pull back from what they are really trying to touch, hold and reach, fearing that it's too late to accomplish their goals. Arthritis is based on a distorted energy, a coiling up of hot energy and a twisting of the human form. It happens to limbs and knees too, but especially hands and fingers, as we reach for things beyond reach, for things we were told as children we had no right to reach for. Arthritis usually happens as people age, although it can attack children, too. It is a holding back of energy instead of a release. We hold on to the negativity in life so that it is unable to escape, which then causes a hot, twisted mess around the part of the body most needed to clasp life and succeed. The inflammation fans the emotional flame as the anger burns up our dreams.

Arthritis also makes it difficult to bend, and bending is connected to flexibility in thinking as well as in physical terms. We feel resentment towards others, perhaps family members who indirectly put a stop to our goals and plans, or towards ourselves because we were too afraid to take chances and have now turned the resentment into self-criticism that has

The Body's Emotional Imprint

caused pain and deformity in the joints. When life doesn't turn out the way we planned it, we blame others, but instead of saying the words we turn the anger back on ourselves.

When someone is close to death, as the body breaks down, the hands often have superhuman strength and cling to anything they can, the edge of the bed, pillows, rails, people. For many the fear of leaving is so powerful and the determination to stay alive so great, that even though the body has already deteriorated, the hands can still retain a vice-like grip. In life we do the same thing if we are afraid to let things go, although we usually use our emotional grip instead.

Problems with the hands and fingers can also clear up just by changing a relationship, getting a divorce or leaving an abusive situation, or by changing jobs or location, and as the fingers are freed from the anger and resentment, we can then grasp the future.

Words

Most of the terms linked to the hand and fingers refer to reaching and clasping or handing something or someone. We talk of giving someone "a hand up," meaning pulling them up, and we also talk of "hand-me-downs" and "hand outs" given to those less fortunate. If we ask others to "take this off my hands," are we really talking about an object or garment, or emotions that have become too burdensome? Sometimes we ask others to "take this/them off my hands," which could be related to a person who have become a problem or a burden that we want to "hand over."

"I can't hang on" demonstrates that the hands can no longer grasp the very thing they are trying to hold. But grasping for life is also a desperate measure as people, things, and jobs slowly "slip away." It is a cry for help, especially when the statement is made about a failing business and the owner "can't hold it together" any longer. Or, maybe the business was a bad proposition and someone "got their fingers burned." Burns, however, take a long time to heal, as do the emotions that go with a wound that's deep, searing and painful, so who was burned and who did the burning? Before fires burn, they smolder for a long time before breaking into flames, so the signs were probably there but were ignored and now that anger has turned inwards.

If "hanging on" refers to health, a family matter or a relationship, and is said by a caretaker, then we should heed the warning as the caretaker may be at the end of their own health, especially if they state that they are at "breaking point" or "clinging by the fingernails." Caring for a family member with Alzheimer's, or someone who needs more care than one can give, is stressful and can lead to a precarious position as the caretaker "balances on a knife edge."

"I just can't seem to reach it" refers to something just out of grasp—or imagined to be out of grasp, as we lose confidence in our ability—like a move to a new place, a change of job, or the end of a project. Other times "we can't seem to reach" others who need help and reject our offer.

Finger joint problems often happen when people are frustrated and let the anger turn back on itself in the form of self-recrimination, gnarling the fingers. When we berate and tell ourselves to "knuckle down" for something we need to do or finish, we usually "put pressure" on ourselves which can cause the energy of the fingers to withdraw and the knuckles to become disfigure.

Sometimes, phrases relating to hands have a positive meaning, as when the young leave home and are "off our hands." Other times it can leave us with too much time as we bewail that "I don't know what to do with my hands," once the offspring, who was the center of attention, has moved out.

What we choose to do with our hands can be positive and creative, or we can "sit on our hands" when we have too much time and too little to do, or don't wish to use the hands for the purpose others think we should use them. It's important to look at the state of the hands to understand how we really feel about the uses we put them to. Are they old, worn, un-cared for, or used, but also taken care of? If we don't value the hands and fingers it's difficult to value what they can do. If we're told enough times

> Hands are to use when we can't find the words.

that we should "give up" on our dreams, then we will devalue the hand that may have taken us there—as a musician, chef, accountant, health worker, activist.

Weakness in the hands reflects a feeling of weakness about our self-image in society. Are we a valuable asset, or do we devalue our occupation and all that it represents? If life has "handed us a lemon" then what do we intend to do about it? Is the feeling one that is "eating away" at us? Lemons are acidic and acid is corrosive, so the body could be feeling acidic and need the pH level balanced, which will help balance the emotions too. Or, we may feel a sourness against another, or they may be the one souring us. Stating "I'm going to take myself in hand" is to recognize that ultimately, we are the only one who can move us into a better position, and doing that will probably alleviate the arthritis too.

See Cuts, Bruises, Feet and Skin for additional information.

HEAD – Face

Basic Anatomy

The head consists of the cranium (skull) and the face. At birth the human skull is made up of 44 bones, but as growth occurs, they fuse down to 22 solid bones—eight cranial bones that fit together at joints called sutures, and fourteen facial bones. The weight of a human head depends of the size of the person but is usually between eight and twelve pounds—the weight and size of a medium bowling ball.

The cranium consists of two major parts, the calvaria (skullcap) and the face, and its main purpose is to protect the brain and sensory organs, the eyes, nose, mouth, and all the muscles, nerves and blood vessels that serve the facial features. The head of a newborn would be unable to fit through the mother's pelvis if not for the fact that the bones of an infant are not yet fused—which usually happens around the age of six years. The reason young children have such large heads and look like cartoons is because the skull grows more rapidly than the rest of the skeleton in order to accommodate the growing brain.

The frontal lobes of the brain, which lie above the eyes and behind the forehead, house the emotional control center and our personalities. They are involved in motor function, problem solving, judgment, self-awareness, impulse control, memory, language and social and sexual behavior—the area where most headaches originate.

The face is the first thing we look at when meeting others as it conveys significant information with regard to who they are, friend or foe, and their emotional and general health, especially of those we don't know. Every line tells a story, as does the shape of the face, skin appearance, bone structure, eyes, nose and mouth shape.

Emotional disharmony

We hold our thoughts in the entire body, but the face expresses them. Here we show love and happiness, stress and sorrow, we smile, we frown, we cry, we laugh. Pain arises in the head to indicate emotional distress. Throbbing aches usually hit just above the eyes, which presents the question of what we are seeing that we don't want to see, or don't want to acknowledge. However, headaches that form a little high than the eye area—mid-forehead—are caused by emotional pain from our thoughts about the past and the present. This area, called the frontal lobe, is the emotional control panel where our pain and suffering lie—as well as anger, frustration, failure, guilt and all the other self-critical words that we use internally. All are bottle up here.

This is the area where personality, self awareness and memory reside, as well as judgment, problem solving and impulse control. Whatever personality traits we dislike in ourselves are lodged here. We judge from this point, beat ourselves up here and connect back to the past, so the pain is very personal and very emotional. This is where childhood memories are stored, which is probably where most of our headaches originate, perhaps from a humiliating or abusive experience that we can't move on from, or words we wish we hadn't spoken, words we wish we hadn't heard, a problem without a solution.

The pain that goes on inside the head is also shown on the face in the form of lines, blemishes, marks, and by the muscles that twist and pull into our own recognizable features. And as the overall face is usually the first thing we notice about a person, followed by the eyes, hair and other facial features, our lives become an open book. The first impression/message from the brain tells us whether we like what we see or not. This is the image we present to the outside, and even though we may look like our parents, or one parent, through gene selection, the looks can change as we get older according to hardship endured, worry, happiness, bitterness and all the other emotions that play out on a daily basis.

Our faces are also formed by thought patterns which produce the emotional framework of the face. Genes may account for some features but they can change when influenced by stress, and strong emotions such as hatred and love. Most of us spend hours in front of a mirror, but how much do we really see of ourselves? Like the rest of the body the face changes every moment—mostly unseen. New mothers right after giving birth, no matter what their age, show a new maturity across the face, not an aging, but an almost imperceptible ripening, a coming of age.

How difficult or easy our lives have been is shown by how rigid or relaxed the muscular framework is. Distorted muscles are produced by the way we have processed words and actions growing up. Weak chins indicate hardship during childhood, while strong chins donate forcefulness, although the forcefulness can come from a harsh childhood that we have steeled ourselves against. Tension in the body turn into facial lines and tension on the face.

The bones in the center of the scalp close up after we are born. This is the outer protective bone that will protect the brain for life, so how secure we feel as the bones close up will show how strong the bones will become, which brings into focus the whole birth process and how we enter the world. How we were handled as we emerge is part of that security, especially as our mother is usually not the first person to hold us. How did we enter the world? After the birth, where did we go? Did we go with strangers into a ward with other babies, or did we stay with our mother in her room? How did others handled us, with loving care or were we roughly treated? What sounds did we hear? All these things are part of our emotional makeup, and part of our health and psychological future. Until fairly recently, newborn babies were turned upside down and slapped to make them cry in order to clear the air passages. What an ignominious beginning!

Usually the right side of the face doesn't exactly match the left side. This can occur from some physical intervention at birth or can develop over time from the way we connect to ourselves and to society. Many of us have a good side that we prefer to present to others and a side we prefer to keep hidden, but is it the male or female side? Or do we feel more balanced on one side than the other? Lopsided faces are usually produced by muscles that pull more on one side than the other, which can give us a lopsided view on life.

Spots and blemishes represent emotional eruptions that we pass through during certain times in life—usually during the teen years—showing parental, school or family problems, peer pressure and all other small irritations that a teen goes through. If they erupt in later life, then ask where the irritation is from: change of job, someone new in the family, a difficult situation that we see as an irritation rather than a large problem, or just a constant stream of irritations emanating from running a home and job. Blemishes also show where there is resistance to doing something, being somewhere, or being with someone we don't wish to be with. Small eruptions, though, can signify that there is something bigger to follow, so what do we really want to say, do, be, that we are not doing? And what problem do we need to take care of now before it becomes a bigger upset?

Facial lines are our life pathways as we travel on. The deeper the lines, the deeper the involvement, which can be positive, but it can also be negative if the lines represent the people and situations we are hanging on to. Superficial lines are shallow and show an inability to connect too deeply to others or to our spiritual side, or we have yet to experience life. Botoxed beauties, however, prefer to hide their pathways as if nothing has touched them.

We take pleasure in babies with chubby cheeks—well fed and happy—but as we age we prefer well sculptured ones to show a form of beauty. Cheeks that are sunken shows how sunk, low and dispirited we feel, through money worries or other problems that are getting us down. Hair that covers the face is usually to hide part of ourselves from public view, or to hide from others, perhaps someone abusive, or from unwanted attention.

Words
Our heads hold our thought about who we are, or who we think we are, and about our past and the emotional pain connected to it. We talk of those who "live inside their heads" as dreamers who store all their hopes, ideas and dreams in their head for safe keeping until a later date, a date that usually never arrives. Things "went to their head" and never left. Sometimes they are misunderstood, other times they are hiding from a frightening world. Those who boast are

considered to be "big heads" as the head balloons outwards with all the ideas that are never released. They know it all, but somehow can't act on what they know, and so, afraid to enter the race, they prefer to stand on the sidelines where it is safe.

A safe vantage point, probably formed from a childhood where accomplishments were never positively acknowledged but the words said to diminish the endeavor became trapped, only to be replayed over and over again. We "feel trapped" as we try to struggle free from the ones who stopped us: an abusive parent, a parent who themselves were never acknowledged? Those who have been abused often keep all their ideas "inside their head" for safe keeping so that the ideas can't be destroyed, away from the abuser who would see little meaning in them.

> Facial lines and wrinkles are the victory signs of a life lived. Botox wipes away the emotional past that formed the indentations.

A "splitting headache" can make us feel as if the brain is being pulled apart, as if there is something dividing the brain into the left and right hemispheres and the conflict is tearing it in two. The home or workplace may be pulling us in two different directions at once. We may feel pulled between our work versus more creative endeavors. Or the family may be demanding too much time, on the one hand, while the boss is demanding time on the other. Or, we may be holding too many thoughts in our head and need to put them into some creative outlet: writing, music, painting, anything that will allow us to express our stored words.

Hoarders often moan, "There's just not enough room," when the real problem is that there isn't enough room in their heads to accommodate all the thoughts that have been stored there:

past hurts, grievances and trauma. The clutter in the mind then becomes clutter in the home as one impedes the other, leaving the problem to compound. Words and actions that seem to by-pass parents as unimportant, are often the very issues that are stored and locked into children's brains, stored until later in life when they turn into stagnating energy, producing a slowing down of the brain function—and a slowing down of physical ability.

Like good clothes that we save for special occasions, we put our "best face forward" in order to give a good impression, and hope that we can "save face" when confronted with something unpleasant. And when we feel good about ourselves we are ready to "face the world" and would much rather be "turning heads" and attracting someone special so that we can "fall head over heels" for them. We also hope that the one we have chosen is "head and shoulders" above the rest—in our culture, height equates with superiority. And in Western society, research bears that out, as taller men are paid more than shorter men.

If we are struggling to "make ends meet," we try to "keep our head above water." The water mark on a boat indicates how much cargo can be put into it, but if the mark falls below the water, then the boat is overloaded and likely to sink, which is how we feel when we we are overloaded. We should note how far under the mark we are, either economically or physically. When swimming, it's also necessary to keep the head "above water" in order not to drown. But water is fluid, and emotions connected to fluid can cause tears that need shedding so that we can "shed light on the subject." What situation are we in that doesn't have enough light on it to show clarity? A money problem that needs professional advice? An acrimonious divorce that needs healing? A severing of

The Body's Emotional Imprint

a partnership? Or are we crying about a situation that has made us feel weak and ineffectual and needs to be "faced." A good cry will usually make us feel better, and may help us find a solution to problems that need releasing.

See Brain, Eyes, Mouth, Nose, Cuts and Bruises for additional information.

HEART – Hypertension

Basic Anatomy

The heart is a hollow, pear shaped, muscular organ about the size of a fist that lies between the lungs, behind and slightly left of the sternum (breastplate). The heart begins to beat 3 weeks after conception and its function is to pump blood in a rhythmic motion from birth to death to all parts of the body. The average human heart beats between 60 to 80 times per minute, although in a well-trained athlete it can be much lower.

The heart consists of four chambers, two on the left side and two on the right, and separating the two sides is a thin, muscular wall called a septum. The upper right atrium receives blood returning from the body and then moves it through the right ventricle to the lungs for oxygenation, while the left atrium receives the oxygenated blood from the lungs and then sends it through the left ventricle to be circulated back around the body. It does this through a series of arteries and veins.

Arteries are blood vessels that take blood away from the heart, while veins return the blood. A series of valves prevent the blood from flowing back onto itself, which produces the sound of a heartbeat as the valves open and close and blood pushes against them to pass through.

The health of the heart can be seen by taking a blood pressure reading, which consists of two numbers, the systole (above) and the diastole (below). A normal blood pressure reading of 120/80 shows the systolic pressure as 120, and the diastolic pressure as 80. These numbers reflect the amount of force the blood exerts against the walls of the arteries as it passes through. Systolic pressure reads the heart muscles as they contract with each heart beat, and diastole reflects the relaxation of the muscles between beats, as the heart refills with blood. The more pressure the blood exerts on the walls, often through stress, the higher the blood pressure number. High blood pressure, represented by higher than normal numbers, is known as hypertension.

Emotional disharmony

We think of the heart as the place where love resides, but it is also where truth rests, and nowadays as many have moved away from family, given up on goals and taken too many wrong turns, many men and women are having heart problems in response to the stress, unhappiness and regrets. We store love in the heart, love for ourselves, love for others, and love from others, and if the heart is functioning well, then there will be a balance between the giving and receiving. A blockage in the heart, though, will also block the ability to receive and give. The left ventricle receives oxygen-rich blood, the right ventricle receives oxygen-depleted blood, so who is giving life and who is taking it away? Do we feel more energized in our female traits, or do we feel that our more male side is having difficulty standing up for what it wants? If we didn't grow up in a family that expressed love, then opening ourselves to receive it can be difficult and can cause us to become defensive and block it out, just as the heart can block the flow of blood. But maybe the one offering the love isn't the one we want to receive it from.

Women didn't have many heart problems until they entered the workplace, and for some it has become a place that is unfulfilling and stifling, forcing many to deceive themselves about the importance of a large paycheck. Women fought hard to enter the workforce, but a number of them are living disappointed lives with little love coming in, and even less love going out. Those who have chosen not to have children in order to continue to work and travel, and others who may not have had an opportunity to have them, often realize in retirement what they missed as they see their friends who do have grandchildren.

In the past many men died shortly after taking retiring from work, often leaving jobs they'd held for their entire working life. Without a job to go to each day they no longer felt important, needed or necessary, especially if their wife had a set a routine that didn't include a retired husband. Many of them died within a couple of years of retirement, and it was accepted that they must have had a weak heart, or held jobs that were stressful or physically hard on the body. In truth, they died of heart problems from no longer feeling valued and from lives that offered few rewards after giving the best years of their lives to work—and little time to the home and family. Once the vitality of life drains away and the blood stops pumping, despair sets in.

The heart is a vital organ which pumps blood around the body by repeated, rhythmic contractions, and once the heart stops then life stop, too, so a heart ailment is usually an indication that there isn't enough energy to push the blood around and keep the body going—or to keep up the pretense that all is well when we are really feeling defeated. Has life played out as we wanted or has it been a life that has turned against us? Many times we live according to the wishes of others and take all the wrong turns but few of the right ones that would have brought greater balance between work and play. Today, the connection between anger and heart attacks has been well documented, but heart attacks are an attack on ourselves, not at the one we are angry at, as we restrict the amount of blood flowing through. Like the damning up of a stream which then traps the water and leads to stagnation. We have a choice about how we live and to what degree we allow others to block our path.

What we feel in our heart flows around the body as it pumps love or hatred into every cell, and those who try to control others, nature, or situations, also try to control their own lives without understanding the consequences of an unbalanced life, a life conflicted as the emotions alternate between compassion and resentment, just as the heart also becomes unbalanced.

In the past heart surgery entailed sawing through the ribcage in order to repair the heart—and the body still carries that trauma—but the repair was really to fix the emotions and enhance the ability to give and receive. Those willing to "open their hearts" afterwards and change their lifestyle have the ability to achieve a better balance, while those who won't or can't, either keep having heart problems, or die. Finding the cause of the anger, resentment and disappointment and then dealing with it will prolong life. So whom have we taken on the anger for, a spouse, business partner, family member, associates at work? Are we disappointed in love, or are we blaming others for our inability to change?

Hypertension is a word we use to describe being "hyper" and having tension. Hyper is overactive and frantic, tension is tightness, strain and stress. It's a little difficult to be both frantic on the one hand and tight on the other, so hypertension represents the two ends pulling against each other like a tug-of-war game. We want to accomplish something, but the tenseness of the situation makes it difficult to do so. Or someone is making us tense and stopping us. Or the situation is so stressful that we are closing down the blood flow, making it difficult to keep the oxygen pumping.

Stress can come from a number of sources: family, work, responsibility, being overloaded with too much to do, money difficulties or marital troubles. Usually the stress comes from what we have put on ourselves as we push harder and harder to achieve, forcing the heart to work just as hard. But are we achieving for ourselves or others? Being hard on ourselves is usually a pattern that is set up by parents, but it can also come from others who push us too hard in later life: spouse, in-laws, parents, boss or coworkers. We bully others—verbally or physically—when we feel inadequate, so if one part of the partnership is pushing and the other one is on the receiving end, the one being pushed will fall, or have health problems. The heart is both the receiver and giver as the blood pumps in and out, so in order to lower the blood pressure, we have to lower the pressure on ourselves.

Words

The heart is one of the most important organs, and so words connected to it carry a heavy weight, just as we have a "heavy heart" if someone very dear to us has wronged us. We are sad beyond belief and from that time on our "heart is just not in it." Despair is linked to the heart as it is a vital organ responsible for being alive, and we feel despair when all hope has gone and the desire to live has gone with it.

When "the heart's gone out of it," we have given up on our dreams and any type of future. The heart/arteries are closing down and we are just going through the motions of living.

The hurts we feel usually come from family members—a parent/child relationship or a marriage—but it can also come from not feeling acknowledged at work or in some situation where we "poured our heart and soul into it" but received nothing back. We may feel that the we helped out from the "goodness of our heart" while others manipulated that goodness to their own ends, leaving us "heartsick" from the sadness that has now stopped us "dead in our tracks."

We can use words connected to the heart for ourselves or others, but the heart is a vital organ, and the words we say today may not manifest until tomorrow, so attention should be paid to those saying the words. Listen to the words of the elderly, especially parents who may be unaware of the message they are sending out. It takes time to block an artery, often years, just as building a barricade takes time, or for a beaver building a dam. A

> The heart is where truth lies -- and it can't be fooled!

blood clot forms when the blood isn't flowing freely, but blood is the force that delivers nutrients and oxygen to cells, and then transports waste away from those same cells. Blood clots happen when the blood stops moving and becomes stagnant. Stagnant pools of water are breeding grounds for insects like mosquitos, which bite and itch. So what, or who, is making us want to scratch the pain out? What would we rather be doing with our time? Who is blocking us from getting there?

Many of us have met people we would consider to be "cold hearted" as they show little emotion to others, only to find out much later that they do have a heart problem. Very often these are the people who have been hurt, or are angry at having to give up their dream to accommodate the dream of others, leaving them "with a heavy heart."

"My heart is broken" indicated that it really is broken, usually over lost love or a love that has passed on, or opportunities that we allowed to pass. The sadness from the event has now produced a broken heart that will never be totally whole again. Often, when we carry "a heavy heart," our actual heart has become too heavy to let the blood flow through it. The weight of a life not lived, not loved, not allowed to have given love—or receive it—weighs heavily, as a life not lived the way we wanted is usually filled with sorrow at what could have been.

When the heart is "broken" it becomes more than one piece, just as the heart is divided into two halves, the right heart and the left heart. Are we bringing fresh blood into a situation or trying to push old blood out? Is one side, or someone, taking over and we resent it, such as "new blood" coming into the business while we are pushed out, or a new partner has arrived while the old one is still fighting over the divorce papers. Or is it a spouse who wants more than we can offer and keeps pushing us to do more, or has pushed us into a job we never wanted? Are we being pushed to take a different direction in our life and the ill health of our heart is sending us that message?

People with heart problems who have aggressive personalities often fight to be heard, accepted and given the power they think they deserve. They feel others have misunderstood who they are, and the more misunderstood they feel, the more aggressive and angry they become. These are the people who tell us to "eat your heart out" or words to that effect, when they want us to envy them. Often said in jest, the words really focus on the need to feel superior, but often the speaker is the one with the heart problem as their anger "gnaws away" at them.

Heart problems also reflect the lies we tell ourselves, hoping that the heart will never find out. These lies include the pretense that we like our job, marriage, family life, single life, and all the other lies that gets us through the day. We may lie and deny the truth but the heart knows. It's easy to fool the head, it's almost impossible to fool the heart.

When we are "doing the work we love," then we are working at a job that fulfills our emotional needs, and we find ourselves feeling "young at heart" as the good feeling fill us "heart and soul." Doing work that doesn't satisfy us will stop us from "putting our heart and soul into it." If the "heart just isn't in it" as we toil away at jobs that are "eating away at us," then sickness will follow.

On the other hand, if we talk of things being "near to our heart" or doing something to "my heart's content," we are obviously doing things that we love. And doing them with someone who is "after my own heart," we have found a kindred spirit with "hearts beating as one" to enjoy life with. These are the lucky ones.

If we "feel pumped" everything is great and the heart is also in good shape. If we "bounce back" after a heart attack, that's even better.

See Chest and Ribs for more information.

HIPS – Pelvis

Basic Anatomy

The pelvic girdle is the bony, basin-shaped cavity in the lower part of the trunk that attaches the lower limbs to the spinal column and contains the bladder, rectum, lower abdominal organs and internal sex organs. It is made up of three bones forming an oval shape and incorporates the lower part of the spine—called the sacral bone—five bones fused into one section which connects to the tailbone (coccyx). On each side of the sacrum are the two hip bones, called the iliac crests, which look like the tips of butterfly wings and wrap around to the front of the body to form the pubic bone, and joining the sacral bone to the iliac crest are the sacroiliac joints. In the pelvic girdle there are structural differences between male and female. The female pelvis is wider and shorter, to allow for childbirth, while the male is higher, with a smaller body cavity.

Like the shoulder, the hip joint is a ball-and-socket structure, called the acetabulum. It is one of the largest weight-bearing joints and allows for the full movement of the leg. Consisting of the femoral head—a ball shape at the top of the thighbone—it rests in a rounded socket with bands of ligaments connecting the ball to the socket to provide stability to the joint.

Cartilage covers the surface of both the ball and socket in order to cushion the ends of the bones and give ease to movement, while a tissue-thin membrane called the synovial makes a fluid that lubricates the joints to eliminate wear and tear. Muscles that overlay the bone structure attach to the abdomen, buttocks, lower back and thighs, all of which help to stabilize and balance the trunk of the body and move the legs and hips.

Emotional disharmony

The hips are the starting point for our forward motion. When we think of walking, we tend to think of the legs, but how we move—with ease or difficulty—comes from the hip joints as we swing our legs forward and backward and out to the sides. At the top of each bone is a layer of cartilage which allows for free motion as the bones slip over each other like a well-oiled machine. If the buffer zone wears away, however, then hip replacement is often performed. The emotional buffer zone for many of us is family and those who love and support us, which is why hip replacement often take place in later life as the support system gradually dies out or falls away.

If the support collapses, through illness, aging, or from too much responsibility, then the pelvic area often takes on the emotions that wear it down. Broken hips are very stressful as they stop movement much more than a broken leg, and are much more serious, usually requiring surgery. The repair, though, is a way to rebuild the confidence that caused the fall that produced the broken bone in the first place. We often break bones in later life when one partner dies and breaks up the partnership, shattering the emotional bond too.

Hip replacement surgery, which has become more commonplace over the years, is also done to repair damage from arthritis, inflammation and stiffness of the joint; rheumatoid arthritis, swollen and inflamed joints; and osteoarthritis, the wearing away of the joint—a painful grinding action that intensifies over time. But any grinding motion in the body represents the grinding down of who we are, the grinding away of future endeavors and the crumbling of the support that we really need to accomplish things. We need strong bones for support, just as we need the fluidity of the cushion between the joints to ease our way. A hip replacement gives people a second chance to ease up and enjoy life a little more, and a good or bad outcome of the surgery depends on how much life we think we have left and how we wish to use it.

Arthritis, rheumatoid arthritis and osteoarthritis, the last of which affects more women than men, is an assault on the joints that we need to move freely. Joints connect two things for strength and movement, and emotionally reflects how we feel about partnering, either one-on-one, in families, in a work situation, or in a group. Do we really want to partner now or are we being forced into a partnering situation such as a business arrangement? Do we want to get married, or stay single? Do we want to give birth to a new project or are we too tired. Do we want to move or are we happy in our present situation?

Joints can connect or disconnect us with family, friends and the things we want to do. We live in a disconnected society, even though technology does much to connect us, but what we really crave is a physical attachment to others who will provide us with support when we need it. Aging often disconnects us from family members as they move, or we move.

Inflammation is caused by anger directed inwards, while we really want to direct it outwards at others, and not being allowed to voice an opinion can put pressure on the joints as the pent-up anger swells to a red hot stiffness and an inability to move. Remaining silent produces anger, which causes inflammable situations, whether in public, as it turns outwards, or in the body, as it turns inwards. A grinding down of

The Body's Emotional Imprint

society by governments will often produce a backlash, caused by feeling powerless, which left unattended will flare into violence on the street.

The pelvic area is also where women give birth, and so how we feel about being pregnant, or becoming a parent, is indicated here. Pregnant women who have lower back and pelvic pain, usually caused by an uneven distribution of the extra weight, is acceptance of the front and back weight and being able to balance the two, like balancing emotions that swing between elation at the prospect of becoming a parent and the fear of the unknown after the birth. Moving into a different life and able to accept a balance between the life they are leaving and the one they are about to enter, and fear of having to take the responsibility for another being. Once they are parents, however, women carry children on the hip bones and so it's a very important area for women both before birth and after. The entire pelvic oval represents the caretaker and the full circle of life from birth to death.

We move towards things we like to do and away from things we don't feel comfortable doing, or that we feel we don't deserve to do. The pelvic girdle gives us strength, and the hip, which cradles the legs, gives us fluidity, so how confident we feel about the future can be seen here. Unfortunately, in this day and age, very few people stride with ease, with the back erect, arms and legs swinging, and good coordination. Usually we walk with the head down and a body leaning forward as into a high wind, as we do battle with life.

Words

Sometimes the words we use for the hips are the same as the ones we use for the legs and feet, words that signify feeling stuck and unable to move ahead, and not being able to "stand our ground" against those who stand in our way. The pelvis is also where movement begins, and so how flexible the legs joints are as they fit into the sockets will indicate how fluid the flow of movement will be from the trunk.

If we feel that life is "grinding us down" then the joints will also be ground down, leaving the body to sink into itself as we allow whatever is "wearing us down" to do so to the point that we become a "shadow of our former self." But who, or what situation, are we allowing to make us look thin, gaunt and shrunken. Or maybe someone else is being beaten down, and we need to take action for them?

The pelvis is a basin shape that is like a protective shell from which we emerge at birth, and the ease with which we appear will affect mother and child into the future. A long, protracted birth can portend the mother's unwillingness to let the child go and the child's unwillingness to leave "home."

Women with "childbearing hips" are considered motherly, while girls who "just want to have fun" are usually slimmed hipped. And women who "swing their hips" in a provocative way and are considered "loose," obviously have hip joints that pass freely.

"I don't think I'm ready for this" new parents often wail as their apprehension creates a division between life before and life after. Or the words may be unspoken but a miscarriage or problems throughout the pregnancy may reflect this apprehension. The duality of wanting a baby but not the responsibility, produces a hesitation on the part of the mother that will interrupt the chance of the baby coming to term.

Women today are conflicted about the timing of having a child, leading many to doubt that they've made the right decision when they do become pregnant. "I'm not sure we made the right decision" implies that this is the wrong time; this can coincides with money worries or anxiety about job security—often two sides of the same coin—or about health problems. Sometimes we break an arm or a leg, symbolizing the conflict caused by unease at the upcoming birth. Or a man's unease can manifest as a pulled muscle at the groin as he becomes unsure about his role as father and provider.

In much of our society, we label women according to their hip width. "Childbearing hips" are usually wide, padded and "motherly," while slim hips represent party girls who just want to go out and play. "Loose" women, on the other hand, have hips that can sashay down the street with the greatest of ease, just like a well oiled machine out for a joy ride.

The pelvic area is also where the genitals lie, so the words connect to our capacity for sexual feelings and how attractive we feel with the opposite sex. Very often, as that appeal wanes after giving birth or with age, so hip problems appear in the form of broken or cracked bones, hip replacement or sciatica—which is pain that travels along the sciatic nerve from the the hip, down the leg, to the ankle—or can show itself as lower back pain. Those with lower back/hip problems talk of "feeling my age." Or they say, "I just can't make it anymore," as walking slows down and there is little will to go much further, or nowhere interesting enough to make the effort.

We also "shoot from the hip" when we want to speak bluntly to someone. But being "hip" also implies being "cool" and cool people typically look good and have an easy gait, as they feel secure and comfortable with who they are and how they are perceived. Hip people are usually seen as young, but hip older people are young at heart with a body to match, so the word is quite literally about flexibility and "going with the flow."

See Spine and Legs for additional information.

JAW

Basic Anatomy

The human jaw consists of two bones. The upper, called the maxilla, is part of the facial bones and holds the upper teeth in place and forms the base of the nose. The lower bone, called the mandible, is the strongest bone in the skull and the only one that can move. Horseshoe-shaped it supports the lower teeth, provides attachment to the muscles for chewing and making facial expression, and forms the shape of the chin. Connecting the lower jawbone to the skull is the temporomandibular joint, a hinge that lies just in front of the ears and allows for the opening and closing of the mouth.

There are twelve pairs of cranial nerves, all of which branch out of the brain, unlike the nerves which emerge from segments of the spinal cord. Some perform motor functions, others have sensory functions and a few have both. The trigeminal nerve, also called the fifth cranial nerve and the largest of them, is responsible for sensation and motor functions such as biting, chewing and swallowing. It has three branches, one to the eye area and the others to the maxilla and the mandible. Most facial nerve pain disorders originate with the trigeminal nerve as the maxillary nerve runs along the cheekbone, upper lip and teeth, and the mandibular nerve passes through the lower cheek, lower lip and jaw.

The facial pain, called trigeminal neuralgia occurs in short bursts and feels like a sharp, stabbing pain that can last from a few seconds to a few minutes. It is so debilitating that it can impact mood, cause sleep depravation, and impede the ability to eat and work. In severe cases it can lead to suicidal depression.

In almost all cases, just one side of the face is affected. Both young and old people can suffer from this pain, although it usually occurs later in life. Often a cause is not found but it may be attributed to age, damage from an accident, pressure on the nerve from a blood vessel, or dental problems connected to teeth or the bite, such as grinding.

Emotional disharmony

How we feel about the food and liquid coming in through the mouth is indicated by how easily the jaws open and close and how wide they can go. The ease with which we can move our jaws hinges on how easily we can open our mouths to chew words before we digest them—or spit them out before we swallow them.

The line of the jaw delineates the shape of the chin, and how far it protrudes or how far it is pulled back is formed not only by genes, but also by our emotional trials during childhood as the facial features formed. How much of a voice were we allowed to have growing up and how freely the words were accepted by the adults around us had a profound effect, especially, if the words were not accepted and we had to draw them back at the last moment for fear of the consequences. As the words were withdrawn, so the muscles followed, pulling the jaw out of alignment.

We may start life with a strong chin, but years of being verbally beaten down can cause the muscles around the mouth and neck to contract, which then pulls the lower jaw back with them to produce a weak chin. Having an overbearing parent, however, can also set the jaw line in the opposite direction, pushing it forward as the teeth lock and the mouth sets into a willful scowl. Many young children do this to indicate their displeasure to a parent when they feel powerless to say what they really want, but done enough times, this behavior will set the jaw line into a confrontational shape. We think of a strong jaw as masculine and powerful, an image that appeals to most men, but in truth it can also represent a stubborn, controlling person who refuses to back down; the reason so many military and political leaders have strong jaw lines.

If the jaw is misaligned, then the mouth and teeth will be misaligned with them. But which side is being pulled, the feminine side or the masculine side? Many today seek chin implants in order to look stronger and more authoritative in their professional lives, but if the weakness is due to feelings of inferiority then the muscles will continue to shorten and will eventually pull the chin implant out of shape too.

Children who were put down for voicing their opinion often have strep throats or other throat problems throughout their lives, as the throat and mouth begin to tighten from a fear of asking for what they want. But it can also happen later in life if those in charge—spouse, parent, partner—constantly belittle us and force us to retreat into timidity. Distortion of the jaw can also happen if children hear angry words spoken by those they love, and not wanting to get caught into their war of words, close their jaws and reduce their words to little more than a mutter.

Silent children who find their voice when older often see the shape of the jaw line change, too, as some of the muscles learn to relax and underused muscles come back into play, allowing the jaw to open wider for a stronger voice. Public speakers, actors and others in authority have strong jaw lines, often from years of training the voice and using the shape of the mouth to annunciate clearly—and being unafraid to be heard.

Nerves that pass from the brain through the jaw also demonstrates how well those circuits are working. As the nerves are the spark plugs that run activity, a severed or damaged nerve will cause that side of the face to stop functioning, indicating an emotional weakness on that side. So who is the fight with, a sibling, offspring, parent? An emotional blockage can cause pain while opening and closing the mouth as the hinges lock at the side of the jaw, but what are the words that are painful to say? Who do we want to say the words to: spouse, children, parents, boss, friends? Are we in a relationship where we feel we can't speak, or staying in a relationship longer than we should have? Have we been silenced by the cruel words of a spouse, friend, or boss, or have we silenced ourselves?

We clench the jaws when we want to stop others from entering, and to hold back feelings of anger, frustration and bitterness as the jaws lock shut, indicating that there is no negotiation. We won't forgive and we won't listen. The tightness of the jawbone will not let words escape or allow new ones to enter, perhaps because of being asked to do something we don't want to do or with someone we don't wish to be with. Or maybe we are the one holding back the words due to guilt about something we've done, or something we are afraid will be found out. Or we hold back the actions of others who have frightened us into silence, such as physical or sexual abuse.

Words

Jabber, jabber, jabber! "Their jaws never stopped!" we say, referring to someone who never stops talking. And today, the chatter never seems to stop. People who talk too much, though, don't usually listen, but is it that others have nothing worth listening to, or that they have too much to say?

Parents often say to their offspring, "Words fail me," but is it because there is nothing left to say or that parents don't speak the same language? Sometimes we "can't find the words to say," or we don't want to say anything for fear of saying the wrong thing. Or, we may be dumbstruck by what others have said, as we exclaim, "My jaw dropped," indicating that we feel astonished by words aimed at us. Or are we in disbelief because we wouldn't have utter the same words, even though we would like to have had the courage? We attack whistle blowers when secretly we wish we had the fearlessness to speak out.

> Even though Sigmund Freud pioneered the understanding of a psychological defense mechanism when faced with unacceptable thoughts, he refused to believe that smoking was the cause of his own cancer. He died of mouth and jaw cancer.

The trigeminal nerve, part of which passes through the jaws, makes it painful to open and close them. The pain, which can be excruciating, can last for months or even years, but it usually occurs when someone is "striking a nerve," meaning that someone pushed a button that caused the pain. As the pain can cause a debilitating stabbing or burning sensation, we have to ask who has the ability to create such pain? Who has that power? Ongoing family relationships where the trouble is never resolved and just keeps on repeating, usually coincides with the pain that keeps repeating. It may subside for a while, but like all family flare-ups it will start up again once the words fly.

What words have been so hurtful that we can no longer bear to hear them? How much pain are we willing to tolerate from the person who pushed that nerve? Or have we said the hurtful words and are causing the pain out of guilt? Would saying what we really want to say help the situation, or make the pain worse? Is there a way to ease the pain—and the situation—so that both parties feel satisfied?

Many older women have jaws muscles set is a semi-smile in order to show the world that all is well—when of course it isn't—but being brought up not to "let the side down," they put on a "brave face." Strokes, which often pull down one side of the body and face, indicates that the facade can't keep going any longer.

People who speak without fear, however, are said to "lead with the chin" as they face any situation with a strong lead. And if the action is wrong, they will "take it on the chin" and accept the consequences.

See Mouth, Teeth and Left/Right side for additional information.

KIDNEYS – Dialysis

Basic Anatomy

The kidneys, dark, reddish brown, bean shaped organs about 4-5 inches long and 2-3 inches wide, are located one each side of the spine near the middle of the back, behind the abdomen.

Their function is to process and purify the blood by removing waste—mostly from the normal breakdown of active muscle tissue—and to aid in the formation of red blood cells. The kidneys also keep a stable balance of salts, fluids and electrolytes such as sodium, potassium and bicarbonate, in the blood. The kidneys filter around 200 liters of blood daily, a quarter of which, once purified, is then recirculated back to the rest of the body, while the extra liquid waste is moved down into the bladder to be released as urine.

If these waste products are not removed they can build up and produce a condition called uremia, which is the accumulation of urinary waste in the blood. When the kidneys fail and are unable to cleanse the blood themselves, a special machine is used for the process called dialysis, which is a life support system—temporary or permanent—that replaces the function of the kidneys with a machine to filter the blood back to a normal balance.

Kidney stones are caused by a mineral crystal formation that grows large enough to block the flow of urine. They are usually formed by a calcium buildup, although stones can also form from uric acid or magnesium ammonium phosphate—usually from repeated urinary tract infections—or from dehydration. They are painful to pass and although the smaller stones can pass on their own, larger ones need to be treated medically, nowadays by the use of a shock waves process called lithotripsy. The waves are strong enough to break up the kidney stone, but can also pass easily through the body.

It is possible to function with only one kidney, which many people do after donating a kidney to a family member or someone else in need, or losing one to disease or an accident. Certain painkillers taken over a long period of time can lead to kidney failure, especially if kidney problems are already present.

Emotional disharmony

The kidneys connect to the adrenal glands and are essential to the urinary system. They represent how well we handle the fight or flight emotions and how we interpret whether an event is a real threat or just an overblown interpretation of it. The decision we make will depend on how well the kidneys are able to filter the blood and move the waste and liquids along to the next stage of the clearing process, and how well we are able to filter the information we receive. Lack of ability to process the information can lead to bed-wetting or incontinence, which we usually link to bladder problems. Weakened kidneys, however, may really be the problem and require attention.

The action of the kidneys is to cleanse and release, especially emotions connected to fear, stress and movement. Here we have the opportunity to cleanse and release our relationships, either by leaving them or by reforming them in a different way that will be more beneficial. This is where we can let go of anything that no longer serves us: working at a job that has taken a toll on our health, living in an environment where we must constantly be on guard about our words and actions, feeling that our escape is blocked by crushing responsibility, or being unable to see a way forward. We have the final chance to cleanse the blood, and ourselves, of all that is no longer wanted or needed. If we don't see a way forward, then kidney stones may form, and how big they become will indicate how secure we feel in letting go.

Kidney stones often form due to dehydration when there isn't enough fluid to flush the stones through, maybe from unshed tears that we have held back from a past event or relationship. Small stones are irritating and can be connected to an irritating person who refuses to leave us alone, a spouse who needs constant attention, parents or in-laws who demand our time, a boss who hands us too much work, or an inability to take time out to process our own lives. Small things have a way of turning into bigger things very quickly, so address the small irritant before it has time to grow.

An over-acidic body can also cause problems with the release of fluids from the kidneys, and this also connects to dehydration. Drinking too little water is a way to deny the body good health, and may cause an inability to release the situation that has caused us to dry up. If we feel bullied by others, we shrink from their caustic words by retreating to safety, but as dehydration affects muscle ability, it will also affect how able we are to remove ourselves from the situation.

We can function with only one kidney, but if the kidneys are no longer able to filter the blood then dialysis is the only option. Dialysis is a desire to become a new person, but needing the strength to make the change. We may dislike the old and what we have become, but refuse to allow ourselves to be satisfied with the what we have, and instead, obsess over what has not worked out. We lack the will to balance our time, money and resources to accomplish our goals, just as the kidneys' filtering function is also out of balance.

But is the right side out of balance or the left? Have we been fearful of someone or some situation for so long that we can no longer function? Has someone overpowered us, even though they didn't intend to? Relationships become unbalances when one person become too forceful and the other side allows it. When we stay in a relationship that has finished, often because of not being heard, then the partnership becomes unbalanced. Are we fearful of getting fully engaging in living? Do we lack the courage to live life on our own terms, regardless of what others may think.

The adrenals sit on top of the kidneys and reflect our exhaustion and fear, but the kidneys are about moving those emotions along, or holding onto them. The decision is ours to take.

Words

The kidneys represent our worries and deepest fears as we deal with the future, our health, money matters, survival and how strong we feel in facing our problems. Feeling that life has been a "waste of time" is to regret that we didn't take enough chances to change its course and have "taken all the wrong turns." We regret being so afraid and letting worry "eat away" at us as we tell others about our health and money concerns, of not having enough put by for future events, or not having the courage of our convictions.

Rain is important for growing food, which in turn feeds us, but lack of water shrivels the plants until they eventually die. Lack of hydration does the same thing for the body as we deny ourselves the emotional watering that we need. Kidney disease—the processing of liquid—is on the rise, which indicates that we are perhaps allowing others to "rain on our parade," stopping any sunshine from entering.

We bathe ourselves to feel clean and fresh, but if we "feel dirty" we then distance ourselves from others, and not allowing the blood to cleanse itself feels the same way. Saying "I just can't process this" is usually about information overload, but the same thing same thing can be said when the blood filtering system breaks down. So what, or who, do we need to confront?

"I've got to move on from this," is the loop inside our heads that won't allow us to progress from a situation that is affecting our emotional state. We often say this after a loss or breakup, but it can also apply to the kidneys if waste is unable to move on too. If we "fear the consequences" and think we've taken a wrong action, then we'll obsess about the outcome, increasing the fear about our circumstances, job, family, and economic situation.

> Mozart died at the age of 35. Sick throughout his life, many have conjectured that the cause of his death was kidney failure. The organ represents anxiety, insecurity and fear -- he lived with financial uncertainty.

When we feel happy about who we are and what we are doing, life "flows" easily.

Fear can also cause us to hang on to people and things that we should cut loose. Parents often won't allow their children to leave, especially elderly parents who fear getting old alone, but the hanging on can also apply to any situation that has run its course. We have to learn how to let things go, whether it's actual clutter or clutter in the mind. When the "blood is pumping" though, we feel "pumped" and ready for action.

See Lymphatic system, Liver, Bladder, Adrenals for additional information.

KNEES

Basic Anatomy

The knee is the strongest joint in the body, and the most complex, as it has to bear the weight of the body while providing flexibility for movement. Four main bones meet to form the knee joint: the femur, which starts at the thigh bone; the tibia, starting at the shinbone; the fibula, at the outer shinbone, and the patella, which is the kneecap. Two joints allow the knee to bend, straighten and rotate slightly from side to side: the tibiofemoral joint connects the tibia to the femur and the patellofemoral joint attaches the patella to the femur.

Surrounding the knee joint is the synovial membrane, which is filled with a fluid that lubricates, protects and nourishes the area, while the meniscus cartilage, a thin, spongy shock absorber, separates and protects the ends of the bones from rubbing against each other and allows the joint surfaces to slide easily. When the knee is injured by a twisting motion, this cartilage is often torn, referred to as "torn cartilage." Keeping the knee in alignment are ligaments, which connect the thigh bone to the lower bones and prevent the knee from making extreme sideways movements.

The largest of the thigh muscles is the quadriceps femoris, a group of four individual muscles that converge at the knee and are connected by a thick tendon. This is the prime muscle for the knee and the most powerful muscle in the body.

Tendons, which attach muscles to bones, join the patella to the lower bones, while the hamstring muscles, which run down the back of the upper thigh and then down the side of the knee, attach to the lower tibia bone. This is the pulley system for the leg extension and bending motion, but overuse or injury to this area can cause tendonitis.

Knee injuries are usually very slow to heal as there are few blood vessels in the ligaments and tendons.

For those who are overweight, every additional pound of weight puts about 5 extra pounds of pressure on the knees when going up and down stairs.

Emotional disharmony

Knees are the midpoint of our legs between the thigh and the ankle. We scrape our knees, fall on our knees, have surgery on our knees and fall to our knees in prayer. Healthy, flexible knees are essential for walking, climbing, sitting and bending, and any weakness will produce a fall, trip or a slowing down of the leg movement.

The action of walking requires the knee to lock as the leg goes backwards, giving us the impetus to propel ourselves forwards. We need the strength to lift, push and stride towards a different location as we move ahead, and any problem with the knees shows a strong emotional connection to anything that requires flexibility, adaptability, and strength. Knees that don't bend and make the leg stiffen, indicates an inability to see both sides of a situation and an unwillingness to bend to see the other side. Stiffness of the knee also shows our inflexibility in life as we refuse to bend to others or resist what others require of us. We may also be pushing ourselves too hard, or into a position we are unsuited for, causing the knee to lock or displace. But flexibility is also required in order to move through life easily, to maneuver turns, take chances and take change in our stride. We need flexibility to deal with problems and to see other perspectives, especially when dealing with the ideas of others who may not mirror our own.

We bend the legs at the knee to get down to a lower level, whether it's to kneel down to children, to garden or to atone for our sins, and the degree to which we are willing to bend shows how yielding we are to those in both a higher and a lower position. A surrender to something greater than ourselves. In religion it shows humility, but a crisis in our faith can also cause the knee to collapse. If the action of kneeling is a chore or is difficult and painful at specific times only, then maybe we are resistant to certain situations or people, or to being asked to take an action at a certain place. Is someone in authority asking for an action that is demeaning? Are the knees a problem more at home than at work? Are we free of pain at the weekends or when visiting the family, or is the pain and stiffness worse at such times?

After sitting awhile do the knees stiffen? Do they stiffen only in places where we feel insecure and with people who belittle us? If there is stiffness, then who is making us rigid? Did our parents have rigid rules that we always rebelled against? Is there a partner or spouse who has rigid, inflexible ideas? When knees stiffen, it is difficult to walk away, so who or what are we afraid to walk away from, or what event or ideas are we afraid to walk towards?

The knees are the shock absorbers for the rest of the leg and require the cartilage and bursa—the small fluid sac around the knee cap—to be healthy so that the bones at the knee can move freely. Healthy knees cushion us from life's ups and downs, and any breakdown here is a fear of the future and and an inability to cope with life in general.

Osteoarthritis is a grinding down of the bone joints as they rub against each other. A conflict, between the two, just as we often feel conflicted between what we want to do versus what we feel obligated to do, leaving life to grind us down as it wears away our will to move away from the conflict. Today, many people have knee surgery, either for total or partial knee replacement, an indication of how much wear and tear the knee has taken and how worn down it has become. As the knee is so important to our forward movement, this surgery replaces our own worn-out piece of equipment with a second chance—a chance to change our thought pattern to a more flexible position. Depending on how that second chance is used, some have a good outcome and are able to embrace life again, while others do not.

Inflammation of the knee is hot emotional pain attached to unresolved anger and resentment about a past or present situation that is keeping the fire alive, making it difficult to participate in life and enjoy ourselves. Who or what is causing the anger that is stopping us? A family member, work situation or past event that was never resolved? Is the inflammation on one knee or both knees? Have we overblown the condition—as in a blown out knee—or is there a deeper emotional problem that needs sorting out, one connected to our chosen path when young? Did we allowed others to chart the course of our life instead of taking charge ourselves? Are we blaming parents for being overprotective, or have we become too fearful to take chances that would change our course now?

Children fall and scrape their knees because they are unsure of the boundaries and move faster than they are able. Most children learn how to deal with boundaries and where the boundaries lie, but those who don't, continue to trip and fall in later years, in business, jobs and decision making. If we felt

The Body's Emotional Imprint

weak at school and so always tripped and fell, then that pattern of falling, and failing, may be imprinted on our muscles and our thoughts, causing weakness in all things throughout life. Perhaps we were constantly told that we would never amount to anything, and now our knee problems in later years confirm that as forward movement slows.

Playing a sport gives confidence, especially if played well, and represents fluidity and agility, but knee injuries from sports denote stubbornness in acknowledging the limitations and a refusal to give in, which then exacerbates the injury. Being overweight presents other problems, as the weight slowly pushes the knee out of alignment. This often leads to the lower legs becoming splayed out as the knees come together to give strength to everything above them. Without intervention, the weight will win out as the walking motion becomes impeded, leading to even less movement.

Words

Knee problems affect flexibility and our ability to maintain a position in word or deed, and if we are unable to bend to accommodate others, then we may find ourselves thinking, "They are so inflexible" without acknowledging our own degree of flexibility. If we are not "carrying the weight" in a situation that requires a team spirit, then we should look at our own actions to see where the problem lies.

Being asked to support others but feeling unable to do so, may be because we are feeling physically weak due to money worries or health problems. We may not verbalize it but being put into a weakened position can make us feel vulnerable and then turn on others, telling them to "take the weight too." Or, the weakness could be a real problem where part of the team really isn't doing enough of the work.

Those who are inflexible, especially the elderly, may be fearful of having to give up their autonomy, although some may have been inflexible in thought, words or deeds their entire lives and getting older just magnifies their rigid opinion. "I have trouble bending," many elderly say, or "I can't kneel any more" implying a lack of faith— probably because their prayers are not being answered—and an abdication of a life that has now become too difficult.

> There are more then 600,000 knee replacement surgeries performed in the U.S. each year. The knee represents flexibility in thought, word and deed!

Kneeling signifies humility, but a fall can be a "fall from grace." "Pride goes before a fall" is said when someone who had an elevated status begins to topple. Many retired people feel this way and start to suffer from knee problems within a couple of years after retiring.

We can also be "brought down to our knees" when we need help but are too proud to ask for it, perhaps because it signifies weakness, vulnerability or old age approaching. The legs may want to move but the knees, which allow the legs to move easily, collapse at the mid point, which as we live longer, also coincides with retirement coming closer to our middle years.

When someone, usually of the opposite sex, make us go "weak at the knees," it implies a sexual attraction. Women used to faint at music concerts, indicating that the men they had "fallen for" made them feel weak and submissive as they gyrated on stage. The knees can also collapse from fear, as the muscles or adrenals weaken.

Wishing to "cut him off at the knees," shows we want to stop an action before it happens, or stop it from happening again. Shattering someone else's knee, called kneecapping, is a method of torture in some countries—it usually damages the nerves and arteries but not always the actual kneecap. It sends the message that they will never have the ability to do the offending action again. They are "put out of commission," usually for life. It is also an action that "cuts them down to size" and forces them into submission as the knees lack the ability to "stand their ground."

See Adrenals, Legs, Ankles and Hips for additional information.

LEGS – Bones –
Osteoporosis

Basic Anatomy

The leg is comprised of three main bones. The femur, a weight bearing bone and the longest and one of the strongest bones in the human skeleton, runs from the hip bone to the knee. The tibia, also known as the shinbone, is the thicker bone of the two bones that run from the knee to the ankle and is also a weight bearing bone, and the fibula is a thinner bone that runs parallel to the tibia. All these bones are connected to the patella (knee cap) and are responsible for movement and for supporting the body's weight.

The leg muscles start at the pelvis, and the act of moving depends on all the muscles interconnecting from the thigh, to the knee, to the lower leg, ankle and then the foot. In order to walk well and have a free and easy gait, all the muscles have to align. Muscles that are misaligned will eventually pull the bones out of place and cause problems in other areas of the body, especially the back, neck and shoulders.

Bones, which are constantly regenerating, come in all shapes and sizes and are comprised of organic and inorganic material. The latter are mainly mineral salts, which give the bone strength and support without bending, and organic bone materials, such as collagen, provide the bone with flexibility. The organic bone matrix is referred to as osteoid.

A cavity in the longer bones contains bone marrow, which usually changes from red—produced by red and white blood cells and platelets—to yellow colored fat cells as we age.

Bone marrow is a spongy, flexible tissue that is responsible for the creation of new blood cells and is a critical part of the lymphatic system.

Osteoporosis is a disorder of thinning bone tissue due to loss of calcium and other mineral components. It results in porous, brittle bones that eventually can cause pain, skeletal deformities and a decrease in height. The elderly are especially vulnerable, but people of all ages can suffer from osteoporosis, especially if too many acidic foods and liquids and not enough alkaline ones are ingested. If the body becomes too acidic (measured by the pH level in the body's fluids), then the blood, which requires calcium to be used by the heart and other organs, will take calcium from the bones. Over time this produces weak and brittle bones.

Women are especially vulnerable to osteoporosis as estrogen protects the bones. At menopause there is a fast decrease of estrogen, when the ovaries stop estrogen production, leading to a rapid bone loss. Exercise, especially weight bearing exercise, is a good way to rebuild the bones, as is Vitamin D—a natural source, of which, is sunshine.

Emotional connection
The legs are connected to how we feel about moving forwards, backwards or sideways, in jobs, decisions, relationships or life in general. We move physically towards goals, things or people that we want, or away from things we no longer want or find necessary. Strong legs, which are our underpinnings and moorings, tether us to our feet and the ground, giving us a grounding for all that we wish to achieve. Loss of leg function is loss of the ability to integrate fully into society.

Leg problems that develop just before a trip, a new job, a marriage or moving to a new place, subconsciously state that we are not sure about making the trip or a fresh start. Children, especially, often develop strained muscles or other leg trouble just before a sporting event they are participating in, translating the fear of failure and desire not to participate in the event, into a physical state. Perhaps they volunteered to save face, or were cajoled into it by parents, friends or peers. Feeling powerful and strong before any event will generate a feeling of excitement at the prospect, any hesitancy is a hesitancy about what the event signifies.

The elderly, who fear growing old and being left alone, often trip and fall as they begin to question their own ability to care for themselves. It can also be a cry to others for support, or an appeal to be rescued and taken care of as the tiredness of having to "stand on their own two feet" begins to take its toll. Falling can also be a subconscious way of getting back at someone so that the other person has to take care of them as they become less able to walk.

The entire human skeleton renews itself continually, giving us all a chance to become stronger and more resilient. Bones are made of minerals, and loss of minerals produce bones that become undernourished, and dry, brittle, and inflexible. Bones give support to the entire muscular system, forming a unit that is strong enough to perform the commands from the brain. Weak bones can weaken the entire body until it collapses. A wearing away of the strength that gave life and the weakness we feel about our place in society. Weak, brittle bones can also make weak, brittle people who can break at any time, or who can also break others with their brittle words. Feeling that life hasn't played fair, they slowly dry up and become sour.

Acidity corrodes as it eats away at things, which is what happens to the bones if they are not well nourished, but it also does the same thing to emotions as the corroding effect produces corroding words that eat away at relationships. Abrasive words can also come from others who chip away, little by little, at our confidence to stop us from doing things we wish to do.

Aches and pains in the leg indicates pain in an emotional situation about stepping forwards, perhaps losing out on a promotion at work to someone less qualified, or a discomfort in a relationship where we are placed in a weakened position with a spouse, sibling or parent. Or being placed in a position at work where a coworker or boss constantly belittle us, weakening our resolve to even ask for a promotion. Or from an unwanted sexual advance by someone in authority and feeling unable to step forward to complaint. If this is the case, then the only options are to either leave or to become more assertive in words and actions. Sometimes quietness is perceived as weakness, especially in a work situation.

All aches have a root cause, and like a tree root, come from a very deep place. When our bones hurt, we are hurt emotionally, and when the bones ache, it is really an ache for all the things we've missed, or no longer have—health, relationships, happiness. It is a tiredness of the soul turned back on ourselves. When the bones no longer form new blood cells in the bone marrow, then we can no longer move in a new direction or do new things with new people.

Many people have one leg a little longer than the other, throwing the position of the hips out of alignment, but in most cases the problem arises at the buttock area where the muscles have tightened. It can also be caused by crossing the same on top leg when sitting, or from one leg bearing more of the weight when walking. Which leg crosses over, the right or left leg, and which one is the dominant side, male or female?

Words

Legs propel us forwards or backwards, and the direction we are going is linked to how much we have to look forwards to in the future and how timid we feel about getting there. As one leg moves forward, planting the foot firmly down on the ground, the leg behind gives the push/impetus to move on. So words connected to the legs are about how strong we feel standing, walking, running and moving—and how far we are willing to "push" ourselves to get there.

Negative words such as "I can't stand it any longer" or "I'm running out of steam," imply weakness—in career, life-style or relationships—while the phrase "I'm making great strides" implies strength and determination in getting there as we "walk boldly into the future" and feel strong enough to endure anything that may stand in the way of our "hitting the mark." If a relationship or job is negatively affecting us, we may think "we don't have a leg to stand on," which immediately has a weakening affect on us emotionally leading to a feeling of powerlessness to take any action.

Being "paralyzed with fear" can be the beginning of a weakness so severe that it will affect mental and physical health as the fear wears away the ability to leave the situation—the legs want to run but the mind can't send the message. Living with someone abusive who has violent mood swings, or working for a boss who is out of control can cause the body to close down, often to such an extent that the muscles will atrophy, producing a type of paralysis. Living in constant fear can have a devastating effect.

Having to "stand alone" is usually said in connection to a decision that is against the point of view of others, while the act of "standing up" to bullies, beliefs, or those who are stronger, is said about someone strong enough to "stand their ground" against them. So how we see ourselves "standing on an issue" or "taking a stand" will show how strong we feel in our ability to act.

Being "stood up," usually by a date, is to be disempowered and dropped, flattened and deflated. So are we "standing" on our own legs, or have we been "stood on" by the action of another. Are they in charge, or are we? Legs are the foundation of who we are and whether we feel we have been weakening by external forces or strengthened by our own inner resources, and whether or not others are willing to give us "a leg up" when we need it.

> Elizabeth Taylor suffered from many medical conditions including scoliosis, hip replacement and numerous back surgeries. A child star from the age of 12, she was never allowed to stand on her own two feet and was never without a man for support.

Legs also affect our athletic ability, and can either keep going for long periods or time, or slow down after a few minutes of exercise. Those who hate exercise often end up in weakened positions in their jobs, as obesity takes over and fewer job choices become available, leading to a downward—or at lease a sideways—position and not an upward one.

If the "rug has been pulled" from under us, then some major event that had a great deal of emotional attachment to it, has not occurred as imagined, such as a job that went to someone else, an engagement that was broken off, a move that will no longer happen. We may have "pinned our hopes" on it, but now that it will no longer happen we feel unsupported, unloved and undone. And if we don't feel supported, then we end up in jobs that keep us on a "treadmill," constantly walking around in the same place. In order to strengthen our opinions, decisions and abilities, and not feel defeated, we need to become more active physically so that we can take a more proactive position at work and move in the "right direction" to what we want. Movement begets more movement.

When we talk of bones and osteoporosis, then we are talking about the foundation that all others things are built on, so feeling "chilled to the bone" or talking of "these old bones" shows how we feel emotionally: cold, old and used up. Loss of minerals produces dry and undernourished bones, and for the elderly it may really be about a poor diet, so even though they talk of their "old bones," they are probably referring to lack of money to buy nutritious food or having the will to cook nourishing meals. Many seniors lack companionship and feel lonely eating alone, but an invitation to eat with others can go a long way in nourishing both their bones and their emotions.

If someone has a "bone to pick" with us, then we know they will find fault with something we said or did. The dissatisfaction they feel about their own lives will be transferred onto us as they nitpick every tiny thing and find fault with everything about us. Nitpickers are unhappy; they can be a sibling, parent, spouse or coworker who feels the need to take others down as their world collapses. So step aside and let them fall.

Things that are not "written in stone" tend to become more malleable, which is how bones should be. Bones are not rigid and inflexible but are able to "give" a little so they don't break. Harmony occurs when we find the balance between being strong enough to "stand firm" and being able to accommodate others by bending a little without feeling taken advantage of.

See Hand/Arthritis, Knees, Hips for additional information.

LIVER

Basic Anatomy

The liver is protected by the ribcage and sits mostly on the right side of the body, with a small portion projecting over to the left above the stomach. It is the only organ with the ability to regenerate itself—unless too badly damaged. Weighing between three to four pounds, it is not only the largest solid organ in the body but, because it secretes a substance, bile, it is also considered a gland.

As a multifunctional organ, it is responsible for the collection, storage and delivery of most of the nutrients in our system, although, only one function, the secretion of bile, is directly connected to the digestive process. Bile, a thick greenish fluid made by the liver, moves from the liver to the gallbladder for storage before going on to the duodenum to play its part in the digestive process.

After a meal, as the food is processed, glucose, amino acids, iron, vitamins and other nutrients are extracted and stored, while at the same time proteins are secreted into the blood stream, and fats are converted into energy storage units to be used at a later time or are used for insulation. Between meals the liver releases glucose into circulation for energy purposes—especially to the brain—and detoxifies chemicals, bacteria, antibiotics, toxins, alcohol and other drugs from the blood, making the liver one of the most vital systems in the body.

A healthy liver makes proteins for blood clotting, which is an important function to stem bleeding. Poor blood circulation

The Body's Emotional Imprint

caused by liver impairment results in inadequate blood clotting and a general decrease in liver function.

Cirrhosis, caused by scar tissue, is a degenerative process whereby fat and fibrous tissue close down the normal blood circulating process, requiring blood thinners (anticoagulants) to stop the blood from clotting in the hepatic portal vein—a major blood vessel that conducts blood from the gastrointestinal tract and spleen to the liver. Cirrhosis is usually caused by alcoholism, but hepatitis, a viral infection which involves swelling and inflammation of the liver, can also interfere with the liver function.

Alcohol is one of the main enemies of the liver as it breaks down the protective mucous barrier of the stomach, leading to bleeding, gastritis and the suppression of appetite, and if left unchecked, alcohol can cause malnutrition. Fetal alcohol syndrome results from the exposure of the fetus to alcohol during pregnancy and is the leading cause of mental retardation in the Western world. Alcohol can pass easily through the placenta to the unborn child to cause delayed development, poor growth during and after birth, heart defects and facial distortions.

Emotional disharmony

Two emotions connected to this organ are at opposite ends of the spectrum: anger, which is often associated with alcoholism, and depression and addiction, which are usually attributed to other causes. But as the liver is related to the blood supply and the extracting of toxins, so the emotions are also identified with the removal system. If the cleansing system breaks down then poisons and other debris collect and form a blockage both within the body and in the emotions, causing outbreaks of anger, self-loathing, resentment, impatience or violence.

If left to stagnate, such emotions can turn inward and develop into depression, which is one of the reasons many alcoholics alternate between being angry and argumentative one minute, and despondent and self-loathing the next. A constant swinging of emotions as they try to find a balance between the two.

On the other hand, since the liver is part of the blood clotting function that stems excessive bleeding, it can imply out-of-control emotions related to freedom, restrictions and boundaries, and finding a balance between lack of rules and limits. The regeneration process of the liver can be a second chance to find that balance for those who choose to take it.

Many who suffer from depression, especially the elderly and obese, who are often too tired to prepare nutritious meals for themselves, may actually be suffering from the liver's inability to perform the extracting functions. Lack of healthful food, combined with a sedentary lifestyle, can play a part in organ failure as the liver becomes overloaded and unable to process sugars and fats, resulting in fatigue, poor digestion, weakness and confusion.

Anger is pain turned outwards, often carried from childhood, perhaps from having an overbearing parent who pushed the child too hard or expected too much too soon. A father who wanted a son to be a carbon copy of himself, or a parent who had to be the life and soul of the party, causing the child to step backwards away from it—and probably the parent too. Unable to come up to such high standards, the child often gravitates later to alcohol and drugs as a way of coping.

The liver contains our addictions and so liver-related health problems usually link to excess: eating, smoking, sex, drug taking and alcohol consumption. If impurities become blocked in the blood, then they find other ways to be released, either through the skin or by gathering at certain points in the body. Acne, eczema or boils, even arthritis, can be a result, as can lumps in the neck, groin and throat, or a distended stomach, although, many with distended stomachs often connect the distention to the stomach, when in fact, the liver enlargement has pushed the stomach forwards.

Words

The words we use to speak about life, often speak much louder about how we are feeling emotionally. Alcoholism and other forms of addiction are an unspoken way of asking for help, but the words used are usually to push others away, "I don't care if I live or die," or, "if I want to (fill in the blank) myself to death, that's my business." These words show a desire to be left alone to self-destruct. We often say, "Why don't you leave me to live my life?" when we push away those we need the most, when what we really want is someone to help us deal with the harmful path we're on, someone who can see beneath the destructive exterior to the small person wailing inside.

Any kind of addiction, whether food, sex, smoking, gambling, is a way of adding something external to lives that have fallen short of what they should have become. Wanting to change reality and unable to do so, we submerge ourselves into something that will change us, and then make the excuse, "I don't have the strength to change" as the addiction does it for us.

When the body breaks down—especially the system that sorts, organizes and clears away the debris—then the will to take action also breaks down, leaving those addicted to cope alone as family and friends fall away. And as the support system crumble, so too do the bodily functions.

Much of recent research has focused on alcoholism being hereditary—genetic—but what is heredity? Most of us at some point find ourselves saying the same words our parents said, especially to our children. We perform the same actions, think the same thoughts, subscribe to the same religions, like the same kinds of foods and follow the same path through life. In other words, programmed the same way as our parents, especially when we say "I sound just like my mother/father" and remember the words that we disliked hearing from them. Or say, "I don't want to follow the same path as my parents" as we see ourselves repeating the same cycle. But our chemical make-up, which is part of our genetic imprint, will also be similar, so in order to change the channel, we need to disconnect the program; different words, different actions, different beliefs, and especially different nutrition.

> Senator Joseph McCarthy, who became chair of the Senate's subcommittee on investigations in the 1950's after charging that communists had infiltrated the U.S. State Department, died in 1957 at the age of 48. The official cause was listed as acute hepatitis, although today it is recognized that he died from alcoholism.

Anyone with a liver problem is really saying, "I'm stuck. I can't move on, even though I want to." And people who are depressed or angry are usually the ones who are least able to ask for the help they so badly need. Blood is the life force that circulates through the body, and liver problems

The Body's Emotional Imprint

are about the inability to circulate freely although we want to. And research seems to bear this out with their findings that many young people who gravitate to addictive behavior do so because of peer pressure, the ultimate terminator of free will as we live more for the opinion of others than for ourselves. Today, worldwide, alcohol and drug abuse among the young is a growing problem, but it is really a cry for some direction in their lives, something to release them from the frustration they feel at not being able to reach out for what they want.

Many children with Attention Deficit Disorder have learning problems, cut class and drop out of school, but they may really be on the losing side of an alcohol or drug addiction passed from a parent, which we tend to ignore when dealing with disruptive kids. Most of them are looking for boundaries, something many have never encountered due to a chaotic home life. They are looking for something that will free them from the damaging cycle they are in. Destructive behavior is a way to escape when there are no other avenues open.

See Lungs, Chest and Head for additional information.

LUNGS – Asthma

Basic Anatomy

The lungs, situated behind the ribcage on either side of the heart, operate as a bellow, and due to sharing space with the heart, the left lung is a little smaller than the right one. Each lung is divided into sections, called lobes; the left lung has two and the right three. The base of each lung extends into the diaphragm, which is a large, dome-shaped sheet of muscle that separates the lungs from the organs below. When we breathe, the diaphragm is drawn downwards and flattens to create a larger space for the the lungs to expand as they draw in air.

At birth the lungs are a pinkish color, but with age they darken into a gray due to inhaled particles and deposits of carbon.

Air arrives in the lungs by way of the trachea (wind pipe), which carries air down from the nose and mouth and then branches off into the left and right lung via the bronchi. Branching from the bronchi are smaller tubes, called bronchioles, which send the air flow into small clusters of tiny air sacs called alveoli. Here oxygen is exchanged for carbon dioxide, a waste gas.

The act of breathing is an automatic action. Once the oxygen—a gas needed in every cell of the body—reaches the lungs, it is moved into the bloodstream and carried throughout the body, while the carbon dioxide is carried back to the lungs and exhaled out. We take between 16 to 24 breaths per minute, although exercise and strenuous activity will increase the breathing rate due to the demand for increased oxygen to the cells. On average, we take about 22,000 breaths per day.

Asthma is a lung disease that inflames and narrows the airways, causing a shortness of breath, coughing and wheezing. When the airways are irritated by external particles, infections or other irritants, then the muscles around them tighten, causing the cells in the airways to make more mucus—a thick, sticky liquid that traps dirt and other foreign matter before it has a chance to enter the lungs. For an asthmatic, the additional mucus is just another layer to narrow the airways and stop the flow of air. When the symptoms are severe, it is considered an asthma attack.

Emotional disharmony

Once out into the world after the umbilical cord is cut, we breathe or cry, taking in air in order to live separately from our mothers. Air is essential to life and lungs are about being alive, being here and taking up space, and so breathing problems indicate our commitment to staying here and participating.

If we feel strong and fully supported, or can support ourselves financially and emotionally, then we breathe deeply, but if we are fearful then the breathing becomes more shallow until we are barely breathing at all, leading to a slow suffocation. But who is doing the suffocating and interrupting our breath? Is it someone or something that is slowly strangling us and halting us from being fully here? Is a situation stifling our creativity and ideas, or is it an imagined fear?

When we are in a fearful state we hold our breath, not daring to breathe until the danger has passed, but if the fear persists, the blood will not be oxygenated enough, causing illness. The anxiety may come from living with an alcoholic parent or partner who has violent mood swings, having parents who have divorced bitterly, dreading bullies at school or work, or worries about money.

Breathing deeply is essential for feeling and functioning well; if we have to labor it then bodily functions will be reduced, lessening interaction with others, which often happens to asthmatics. If the initial problem isn't dealt with, then lack of physical activity can lead to obesity, depression and a closing down of future endeavors and goals—just as the lungs close down on oxygen.

As we exchange oxygen for carbon dioxide when we breathe, so we sometimes need to exchange negative people and situations for more positive ones in order to stay healthy, so what is not being released that should be, a marriage, an adult child who we have come to depend on, a job that we are afraid of losing? Or have we lost someone we did depend on who left us unprotected financially and strangled with debt? What stifling situation is causing the inability to breathe with ease? A situation that we don't want to confront, or someone we are afraid of confronting?

The lungs also represent grief, caused by a death, tragedy, or an emotional ending to a long relationship. Deep sorrow that isn't dealt with eventually takes away the will to live, or the will to breathe. A shutting down of life that can happen at any age.

Asthma is a chronic disease that affect the ability to take in air, and once the airways become restricted with too little air passing through, then panic attacks can occur. Airways become smaller as the muscles tighten, giving the sensation of being choked. But who is trying to strangle us? Is it a situation at work or at home, or a person who is cutting off our air supply? A husband or wife demanding too much, a boss

The Body's Emotional Imprint

who expects more than we can deliver, a situation at work where we cannot voice our opinion but wish we could? An abusive situation where we are not allowed to have a voice?

The number of asthmatic children has increased over the years and we blame the quality of the air, along with many other things, for the increase, but we should also look at the home life of these children to see what has unbalanced their emotional stability. Are they happy, do they feel secure, are they in a stressful situation? Do they have panic attacks when separated from a parent? Are they placed in violent situations on a constant basis? Asthmatic children are often sensitive to family situations around them and may take on the fear of a parent who is trying to show strength in a distressing situation; a parent they love or fear losing.

Asthmatics make wheezing sounds, gasping for each breath as if it will be their last. A panic at being left to cope with life alone, and with the situation they are in, but also knowing that they can't change things. We think of allergic reactions as coming from certain foods or airborne particles, but an allergy is an irritation, so we should look where the irritant is coming from. The world has become a frightening place, and when we take our first breath, once out of the safety of the womb, we are separating ourselves from our mother and becoming independent. As many parents now work long hours at their jobs and their children are in the care of others, it leaves some children distressed and vulnerable without a parental presence.

Shallow breathing places pressure on the system since it doesn't provide enough oxygen for the blood to circulate freely, just as we have placed restrictions on the environment, leaving both humans and the environment suffering from the same thing—lack of clean air. Many elderly have shallow breathing as their bodies begin to hunch over, giving the lungs less space to take in air and leaving them with a feeling of life pressing inwards. Smoking, too, closes down the lungs until they no longer function and the person dies, but smoking is addictive and ultimately is caused by feeling disconnected in society. Lack of self-confidence translates into lack of ability to stand our ground with others who may be overbearing and smothering as we fight for space. A fight to be heard and given a voice, and to know that we have enough air to make ourselves heard. Smoking is a slow suicide—even though most smokers would deny it.

Words

Words connected to the lungs are not only about air, but space too. "Give me a breather," we say when we need tangible space or time away from a work situation or a relationship that has become smothering. "I felt as if I couldn't breathe" is an indication of someone closing down our air supply, probably because they require our share too. They often have enough of a voice for two people, while our own becomes less important. When we speak of "feeling suffocated," we may feel a crushing weight on the chest that leaves us unable to escape the person or circumstances.

On a more positive note, we also speak of someone being "a breath of fresh air," someone with fresh ideas, looks, personality; anything that brings a new perspective to a situation. They allow us to "draw breath," see things in a different light and bring lightness into our lives. It is what fresh, clean air is supposed to do to our bodies as it clear out the old, stale and worn and brings in the new.

If we manage to escape a "suffocating situation" we want to "fill the lungs with air" instead of "holding our breath." Holding it until what, or who, has gone by? A person who won't allow us to breathe freely? Someone who dictates our lifestyle and the words we say and the actions we take? We hold our breath when we are fearful, "not daring to breathe." When we are anxious in a relationship, we are apprehensive as we try to gauge the other person's emotions, trying to avoid a temper tantrum that can flare up for little reason. We label them "blustering bullies" as they suck the air out of a room and leave in their wake a trail of destruction, much like a hurricane.

Babies and small children "shout at the top of their lungs," sometimes because they are in pain, other times for attention, and adults do the same thing when angry. We respond with caution to people who shout loudly as it can lead to an unsettling condition, even if the words are directed at others. Powerless

> We associate lung cancer with smoking, but many who die of it don't smoke. The act of breathing necessitates inhaling the positive and exhaling the negative, but if one side overwhelms the other then an imbalance occurs. Lung cancer is about finding that balance.

men in domestic disputes, usually husbands who have jobs with little power, take it out on those who have even less, their wives. Shouting can escalate to out-of-control actions that takes the form of confrontation, especially large groups gathered for a common cause; street protesters who voice their anger as they take aim at those in higher positions, union workers demanding to be heard.

Some children use holding their breath as a way to hold their parents to ransom after demanding, "I want that" or "I won't do it" until they get what they want, and as holding the breath can eventually lead to lack of oxygen to the brain, parents usually acquiesce to their demands as a brain dead child is even more trouble than a demanding one.

Words of panic or danger, phobias or feeling nervous lead to shallow breathing, depriving the body of enough oxygen to feed the muscles to make them stronger in order to face the danger. Children don't use words to describe how they feel, but do make excuses for not going to certain places or with certain people. Usually this is a warning to parents to look for the real reason behind the excuses, such as bullies at school or unwanted sexual advances, or peer pressure. Or, the excuses may be linked to real problems with breathing which can cause panic attacks.

Healthy lungs and deep breathing show an ability to deal with whatever life throws our way—and feeling strong enough to deal with it. So any problem with breathing indicates that there is something bothering us with regard to our safety, whether it is fear of losing a job, a home, relationship, or just being fearful of living day to day. Being a news junkie can also cause us to overload on the negative and push out the positive—just as the lungs become less able to take in enough oxygen and are not capable of letting go of the destructive carbon dioxide.

See Liver, Adrenals for additional information.

LYMPHATIC SYSTEM –
Tonsils

Basic Anatomy

The lymphatic system is a circulatory network of ducts and nodes that transport a clear fluid called lymph, around the body to help balance fluids, remove excess waste and fight infection. This fluid, which penetrates almost every tissue of the body, is distributed through a network of tiny lymphatic vessels as skeletal muscles pump the fluid through. A series of valves prevent the fluid from flowing backwards. Fluid and plasma proteins that leak out of tiny blood capillaries are collected by the lymphatic vessels and returned to the bloodstream. Without this activity, fluid would build up in the tissue and edema—severe swelling—would occur.

The filtering process is performed by lymph nodes, small, kidney-shaped organs that form in clusters, mainly in the neck, armpit and groin. There are around 600 lymph nodes in the average human body, and each one is filled with many lymphocytes, white blood cells that help protect the body from infection. Macrophages, which occur in almost all tissues of the body, start out as white blood cells and engulf and digest cellular debris and pathogens, stimulate lymphocytes and other immune cells into action, and help to heal wounds. The filtered fluid then goes into lymphatic ducts, which carry it back to the blood supply to be recirculated.

Because one of the main areas for lymph nodes is under the arm, many believe that tight bras can cause constant pressure on the breast tissue and impair the circulation of the lymphatic system, causing toxins, bacteria and other debris to become trapped. Over time, this fluid buildup can cause breast-pain, cysts, or even cancer. This underarm area is also where deodorant is used, often with cancer-causing ingredients such as aluminum.

The lymphatic system is a passive drainage system that lacks a pump of its own to push the fluid through, so it flows via breathing, exercise, movement and massage, and the slightest constriction will inhibit the lymph flow and cause congestion.

The tonsils, situated on either side at the rear of the throat, are comprised of soft lymphatic tissue, much like lymph nodes, and serve to trap and fight infection coming in through the nose and mouth. When infected, the tonsils swell and become inflamed, causing a sore throat, fever, or pain when swallowing. Left alone, they will usually shrink back to normal size, although some doctors recommend surgical removal, called a tonsillectomy. Today, there are fewer tonsillectomies than in the past as the tonsils are now recognized as part of the immune system.

Emotional disharmony

The lymphatic system is the delivery and pickup service for the immune system as it fights invaders, clears debris from the blood and drains excess lymph fluid. A failing lymph system leads to stagnation and drained energy. How well they all function indicates how well we will respond to the invading parties and how protected and energetic we feel in dealing with them. The system gives us the ability to move freely with few restrictions placed on us, by others, or by our own fears.

An exhausted lymph system indicated that we have weakened our defenses, perhaps by not being able to repel those at work who try to stop our progress or by not having the courage to demand what we want . When the immune system breaks down it leaves us vulnerable to others who are opportunists and take advantage of our weakness. Lymph nodes are found singly or in groups, so is the problem related to an individual or a group? Those who invade our space can represent a never-ending stream of annoyances that we have to fight in our daily lives, a job that demands too much of our time, a need to protect privacy online, being forced to accept a cut in pay, bills that are the wrong amount—but never in our favor—causing us to backtrack on things that should have been done but never were. All small things that collectively wear away our resistance.

Tonsils trap bacteria and filter out irritations, but if they become inflamed, then it implies anger and irritation from others—usually parents—that has become trapped. In the past, once removed, all the words that needed to be spit back out were, instead, forced down the throat with nothing to stop them, no gatekeeper to keep them out. Now the words had to be swallowed.

Hoarding is all about not clearing out the mess and being able to clear out all unwanted "stuff." Many hoarders have health issues, especially allergies due to an accumulation of dust, but they also trip and fall as the clutter impedes movement. But how well do we want to clear up our lives, and the emotional mess that caused the clutter to accumulate in the first place. Do we want to get rid of someone we just can't let go of even though the relationship is over? Or is it parents who won't let us go, or parents we will not allow to leave. Clearing up the planet is really a need to clear up our own mess and health problems. We desperately want to be healthy, but find it increasingly difficult to do so given all the toxins and poisons we take into our systems, and as the planet becomes overloaded and clogged, so too, does our lymphatic system.

Lymphatic cancer, called lymphoma, is our inability to deal with all the irritants of the day and the curtailing of our freedom. Feeling vulnerable and weak, we turn the disease back on ourselves, perhaps by not speaking up for our rights, or feeling responsible for others when we would rather be free. Hodgkin's lymphoma is a cancer of the lymphatic system which can spread beyond the lymphatic framework to others areas. Spreading beyond the boundaries imposed on it, and us.

Words

Because other parts of the body are better known than the lymphatic system, we tend to understand them better, but if we talk of wanting to clear things up, or fight those who don't have our best interest at heart, then the words may connect to this cleansing system. Very often the words relate to our work as we say, "Let's clear up this situation once and for all," or "I want to get a clear idea of what's going on here." We know there is a problem but are not sure where it originated or how to really get to the bottom of it, but we also know that without action the problem/cancer will spread.

The problem could be connected, quite literally, to the environment and the food supply. Air quality in the workplace may also be making us sick, especially now that we work in high rises where windows can't be opened. Problems with the lymphatic system are about not having the resources to fight back, either politically, physically or emotionally.

Feeling "stuck in a dead end job" will lead us to stagnate in life and in health, as a blockage stops our progress and allows the

The Body's Emotional Imprint

frustration to grow. We want to move on, but the job market, family obligations, or some other reason, dictates that we can't. And just as the debris in the body collects in one particular place, so our words can also relate to where the nodes cluster, in the groin, neck or armpit as we vent that the boss, or someone else is a "pain the in the neck" or we blame others for "poisoning the workplace environment."

Problems in the groin connected to sexuality and the functioning of the genitals, but the real problem may be one of not allowing the negative emotions to flow around the body and out. We may feel that someone is too demanding sexually and we are not able to release the build up of negativity connected to that insistent person, or there is a buildup of past words that were promised but never acted upon—a marriage, divorce or separation. A relationship may have soured, and we now want to " get clear of him/ her." But who is responsible for the buildup of negativity? Who has allowed the emotions to bring down the relationship/immune system? If someone else caused the problem, then we should move beyond the situation before it grows cancerous.

> Jacqueline Kennedy Onassis, widow of President John F. Kennedy, died from cancer of the lymphatic system. Even though she lived a healthy lifestyle, she couldn't protect herself, or fight back, at the wagging tongues when she married Aristotle Onassis.

If we have a low immune system and catch every cold and virus, we say, "I just couldn't fight it any more." But what is the fight against, a bad partnership, marriage, demanding people, money problems that are eating away at our resources? Does the body need "clearing out" as in a detox, or do we want to clear ourselves out of a situation that is making us ill. Or do we need to clear someone else out so that we can cut the cord on the responsibility of having to care for them: a sibling, aging parent, or someone we no longer love, need or want in our life.

See Neck, Genitals and Breasts for additional information.

MOUTH – Teeth

Basic Anatomy

The mouth is the oral cavity that includes muscles, glands, the hard and soft palate, teeth, tongue, cheeks and lips, that collectively enable us to speak, chew food, take in liquids, breathe, taste, and look attractive. The mouth is the origin of the digestive tract, where teeth and the salivary glands, which secrete chemicals called enzymes, aid in breaking down food and guard against infection.

Just behind the mouth is the pharynx, a single pathway that serves both the respiratory and the digestive system, Saliva kills bacteria and keeps the lining of the pharynx and the mouth moist, making it easier to swallow.

At the roof of the mouth is the palate, which separates the oral cavity from the nasal cavity and is divided into two parts, the hard palate at the front and the soft palate in the back.

The tongue is a muscular pinkish organ anchored to the back of the mouth by tough tissue which allows for swallowing and speech. Tiny bumps called papillae cover the tongue, giving it a rough texture, and coating this surface are thousands of taste buds which connect to nerves that run into the brain to transmit taste signals. There are four common tastes: sweet, sour, salty and bitter.

Lips, which encase the mouth and contain receptors along the surface to help determine texture and temperature, are usually colored a red to reddish-brown because of blood vessels close to the surface of the skin.

Cheeks, which we often don't associate with the mouth, have a thin layer of fat just under the skin, and facial muscles under the fat layer. These muscles help to maneuver food around in the mouth, assist in the formation of speech and create facial expressions.

Teeth are hard structures in the upper and lower jaw that not only chew foods, but also give shape to the face and aid in speaking. During a lifetime we have two sets of teeth. The first ones—the primary teeth—appear between the ages of six months to three years—and are then slowly replaced by the permanent teeth—which should last a lifetime—after around age six. These primary and permanent teeth help form the shape of the jawbone.

Emotional disharmony

The mouth represents how we feel about speaking, kissing, taking in food—nourishing or otherwise—and liquids. We speak through the mouth and how well we enunciate our words indicates how authoritative we feel and how secure we feel in our opinions. If we were constantly put down for our opinions when young, we learn to retreat, which is what the mouth does as the muscles pull back and the mouth slowly closes, producing mumbled words. The mouth is about how authoritative we are in relationships, especially in a marriage, but it can also relate to any relationships, such as in business where we may have "little say" in the running of it.

Older women tend to form the mouth into a set smile, giving nothing away about their real problems and hurts, but pulling the muscles of the mouth back is really to suppress the words they want to say. Often, they are married to men who are forceful both in business and in the community. When muscles foreshorten, they contract and distort, which disallows the full length of the muscle to form, just as their opinions or their creativity is not allowed to form, or the ability to allow life to form into something that is wanted.

Food is also connected to our growth—in stature, status and emotionally. How we think of food is more important than the food itself, which can nourish our emotions or make us feel impoverished. Anorexics deprive themselves as a way to take control in an otherwise controlling relationship. We deprive ourselves of the nourishment we need to live well when we feel undeserving of good things. Obese people overeat as a way to feel self-love and to compensate for love and other things they feel cheated of—a happy childhood, beauty, popularity, a wealthy family, or parents who spent time with them.

We can choose to sit down to meals and serve good food in a pleasant situation and with happy people around, or we can serve meals in a mad rush, where the family never sits down to a meal together and food is something to gulp down before leaving the table quickly. Were meals rushed, with no time to talk to parents, or were they pleasant events where opinions were valued? How we first perceived food will eventually dictate our meal pattern into adulthood—unless we understand the emotional imprint that was stamped onto us as the food was served.

Lips are sexual and for kissing, and women take power by wearing lipstick as a sexual sign and bite their bottom lip or pout and pucker their lips as an invitation, but blisters on the mouth indicates that we don't want to kiss the person or people involved, a way of sending an external message to keep them at a distance. We also shout, whisper and sing with the mouth, and when we need to feel in control of a situation we set the mouth in a defiant position by closing the lips tightly. When we curl the lips inwards until they disappear, we are holding back words in a relationship where there is no acknowledgment for who we are or what we have achieved, leaving others to overshadowed us.

Sores and other small eruptions on the mouth are an indication of anger. Canker sores inside the mouth signify words that need to be said but are still contained, while those on the outside suggest words still hovering, not quite said but hinted at. We spit out things that are distasteful and we spit out words in haste. Herpes on the mouth usually appears after a bad relationship or a sexual one that left us feeling used.

Bad teeth and teeth that decay and fall out reflect the desire to drop the decaying relationship or lifestyle that has caused it. We often blame sweet foods for the decay, but sweetness that isn't swallowed will stay in the mouth to cause decay. Plaque does the same thing as it adheres to the edge of the teeth, preventing them from staying clean and healthy as it clogs the gum line. It forms where the hard tooth meets the edge of the softness of the gum. In a healthy mouth the two will meet, with the tooth visible while the root—where emotional problems begin—is covered. Decay usually takes years to appear, and so the event that triggered the tooth decay may be way back in the past.

Gums hold the root of the tooth in place and problems here pertains to rootlessness. How rootless are we? Do we move around a great deal? Did we live in a great many places as a child? Was moving an upheaval? Were we unable to make friends, put down roots and have relationships? Once the gums become infected the teeth become loose and usually fall out. Gums represent how safe we feel speaking and smiling, and how protected and secure we felt as a child. Healthy gums show confidence—even if the teeth are capped or false. Many elderly people have loose teeth or teeth that have fallen out, as they feel insecure and unprotected as they age.

When we go to the dentist to have a tooth removed, it is ripped from us and is a violation of the mouth. Any problem with the mouth, gums and teeth is an indication of timidity about speaking our mind, and showing our presence, whether at meetings, at work or in the home. We may be afraid to sink our teeth into things that we feel are beyond our capabilities, or are afraid to put our opinion forward, fearful of what others will say.

Chewing breaks down the reality so that it can be swallowed, but bad teeth in kids usually indicates bad family relationships, and even though the food they receive may be good and nourishing, the emotions are not.

Grinding the teeth down is a way of harming the very things we need to chew our food; grinding them down so that we are unable to receive the sustenance we need. Feeling guilt or anger at ourselves for something we said, the grinding action is an act that we do in our sleep, when the subconscious is up and running and we are not. A reminder to pay attention when we do awaken and to deal with the problem, people or emotions that are causing us to want to grind the problem down and out.

Words

The mouth represents what we want to expose of ourselves to the outside world. The muscles around the mouth can either pull it back into a smile, down into a frown or hold it in a rigid way so that few emotions are allowed to pass. Many people, especially women, hold their mouths in a set semi-smile in order to give the appearance that all is well—when obviously it isn't—and women who endure unfaithful husbands but still stay in the marriage, usually have frozen smiles in order to "save face." These women also botox the lines out of their foreheads in order to look young again so they can compete against the younger women the husband is chasing. Then they "grin and bear it," although the same can be said for anyone who stays in an abusive situation, at home or at work.

Normally the mouth tips up or down at the corners, but it can change direction if the muscular structure changes. Too many unhappy events and the mouth will set into a depressed look, but long term-happiness can move the direction upwards.

Passionate kissing burns about 2 calories a minute, which is a little more than the 1.3 calories burned while laughing.

People who talk of being "down at the mouth" have lost all joy in their lives. The word down in any context is to go in a downward direction, and in this case has either emotional or health implications, perhaps referring to a job or a relationship that is "going downhill." The word "down" can also indicate heart problems, as research has found a link between gum problems and the heart, and without joy in our lives and others to share with, we often don't have "much to smile about."

We may know people who are "close mouthed" and who don't give much away verbally, but the reason for the closed mouth may vary, from business dealings to living with sexual abuse; it may really be hiding secrets that they want to talk about, but dare not. Kids, on the other hand, are often "close mouthed" when they are doing something they don't want their parents to know about—taking drugs, dealing with a bully, feeling depressed, or having problems with school work. If someone has "words put into their mouth" it implies someone stronger who is getting the upper hand. So check out your children's peers and those they are hanging out with.

If we feel "fed up to the teeth," then we are fed up to the core of our existence, as once the teeth fall out there is nothing to use to break down foods as they pass from the outside to the inside. We may feel a lack of support and encouragement at work or from the family. When we don't receive enough validation for what we are doing, then we tend to drop out of society, just as we do when teeth fall out of the mouth, but as fixing teeth requires money, the support needed may really be economic.

Politicians and others who are out to impress but do little in the way of action, are called "big mouths." They are said to "talk out of both sides of their mouths," as they cover them-selves from all sides, and they are not to be trusted as they "run off at the mouth" without saying anything substantial.

The colon is connected to the actions of the mouth as it is the opposite end of the digestive system, the place where the remains of meals are evacuated. The mouth is the place where "bullshit" originates as the words are spoken and then have to be processed, but living with someone who con-stantly fabricates the truth can eventually cause health prob-lems as we try to "second-guess" the words as fact or fiction.

Teeth tend to have a negative connotation. We "grind our teeth" when we are nervous or fearful, and "clench our teeth" when we are angry at someone but not allowed to express it. The opposite is to "show our teeth" to indicate to others that we are angry and will no longer accept their treatment or words. Dogs show their teeth when ready to attack. The act signifies aggression and anger, which could also be connected to a liver that isn't functioning well or to toxins and bacteria going from the teeth and gums into the gut to cause digestive problems.

We "cut our teeth" on new situations, just as we begin to chew real food when we get baby teeth and leave mother's milk behind, so problems with teeth and gums may come from a desire to separate from a parent, or with parents who won't allow a separation, even when the child is older.

Sometimes it is the words not spoken that say the most, and adults who were silenced as children often make up for it in later life. They are the ones who lead revolutions, advocate emancipation, march against wars, rail against atrocities and point out inequalities. They are the ones who process what they see, but keep silent until they have a chance to voice their opinions. They often become great leaders who change laws, society and influence matters of justice.

Gums hold the teeth in place and are the moorings of both the teeth and how we feel about our place in society or the situation we are in. Gingivitis—severe gum disease—is caused by bacteria of the gums, which if left unattended will result in the loss of one or more teeth. But we need teeth to eat and chew our food and be able to "sink our teeth" into something." Perhaps a project or job to make us feel that we have some worth, or a project that will absorb us. Or we may wish to literally sink our teeth into someone who is taking away our ability to do something we want to do. Someone who makes every action we take so difficult that it seems as if we are "pulling teeth" in order to make it happen, someone who leaves a "bad taste in the mouth" by being uncooperative. On the other hand, we may be the one wanting a "tooth for a tooth" which can eventually, through a constant nagging desire for revenge, cause our own teeth to fall out.

There are many words and saying about the teeth as they are very important to the quality of our lives. Teeth give us confidence to smile and to enable us to take in nutrients from food to nourish the body and brain, but when we speak or hear words connected to the teeth we should also check that there are no hidden problems in the gums ready to erupt, just as we may be ready to erupt at someone.

See Neck, Throat, Stomach and Colon for additional information.

NECK – Throat

Basic Anatomy

The neck is the bridge between the head and the body—thought and action—and is one of the busiest network in the body, as foods and liquids are swallowed and air moves in and out as respiration takes place. It is where the muscular system supports and connects the head to the body, and also protects the nerves that carry information to and from the brain, which, even though it comprises only about 2% of the body's weight, requires 15 – 20% of its blood supply.

Passing through the neck are veins, arteries, muscles, nerves, the esophagus, vocal cords, the larynx, trachea and part of the spinal cord. Several muscles of varying lengths and thickness support the neck and enable it to turn and swivel, while carotid arteries supply the head and neck with oxygenated blood and the jugular veins bring deoxygenated blood from the head, brain, face and neck back to the heart.

At the top of the spine is the cervical spinal cord, which is surrounded by vertebrae for protection, while ligaments stabilize the vertebrae to allow the nerves to send messages to and from the brain. Lymph nodes, which drain impurities out of the body and play a role in fighting infection and bacteria, are also located in the outer neck area.

The throat, a ring-like muscular tube which lies behind the nasal cavity in the neck, channels food and liquid down to the digestive tract by way of the esophagus, and air into the lungs through the trachea (windpipe). When we swallow, a flap called the epiglottis moves across the larynx to keep food out of the windpipe.

The larynx, better known as the voice box and vocal cords, moves air that we inhale through the nose and mouth down the trachea into the lungs, and moves air that we exhale in the opposite direction.

Topping it all off, quite literally, is the thyroid gland, which wraps around the windpipe at the front of the neck and helps regulate the metabolism.

Emotional disharmony

The neck is the bridge between the external and the internal, outside reality versus inner needs. Everything that comes in through the nose and mouth passes through the neck, so the type of foods and liquids and quality of air that we take in will affect the health of the entire body. And how clear the air is, and how good the food and liquids, indicates how clear our intentions are about being here.

If swallowing food becomes a problem, or food becomes stuck in the throat, then we should look at what are we being forced to swallow that we wish to reject. Who or what is forcing us to choke on something that we find unacceptable. And where were we when we started to have difficulty.

Coughing is an emotional irritation that manifests as a physical one and can be connected to either the throat, neck, or lungs. A superficial cough is trying to release something or someone from the neck/throat area, but if the cough goes deeper down into the lungs, then the irritation also goes much deeper. Someone at home or work making too many demands, or a rift with other family members or coworkers which is causing unease? Coughing signifies that we want to eliminate an irritation that we have allowed to go down too far, something that should have been taken care of in the past, but wasn't.

A cough can also produce mucus, which drains down the back of the throat from the nose, or comes from the lungs, so is the irritation coming up to clear, or going down further to develop into a major health issue, such as fatigue, chest pain or breathing problems? Is the irritant being taken care of, or being pushed further down in the hopes that it will take care of itself? Or are we being pushed down in life by someone stronger, physically, verbally or economically.

The throat and neck are also where our air supply flows and cutting off that supply leads to death, so difficulty here implies a problem with living, being here and participating in life. On the other hand, if we want to strangle someone, then we need to look closely at that relationship. Maybe what we really want to do is to end the relationship. But what were the words or actions that prompted such a violent response? Any action directed at the neck implies that the effect will be negative and hurtful as it damages the relationship between the head and the body. If we want to do the action to another, we should be sure that we won't be on the receiving end later on, so we may want to find a better way to deal with the problem before it gets out of hand.

A stiff neck implies a rigidity in thinking, seeing in one direction only as we reject any other opinion than our own. This eventually leads to narrow-mindedness as the neck muscles constrict, and conflict arises when neither party is willing to see the other side. Many workers get stiff necks from a particular person at work who is stubborn and isn't a team player, or from a boss who is unbending in their demands. We put the blame on the way we sit at the computer, but it may really

The Body's Emotional Imprint

be that we are putting our neck into an unnatural position in order to move away from the offending party.

Constant sore throats represent a constant sore point in our life, something that we haven't dealt with, or don't want to deal with, or something that at this point can't be dealt with. We tend to get sore throats before an important event, such as giving a speech, making a decision that involves talking to another—usually someone who is unavailable emotionally, or someone we are worried won't agree with the decision we want to take. We may also lose our voice because we are too afraid to speak up, or don't want to make a commitment.

Throat cancer is related to having a voice and being heard, and often people who work with words in the public eye— actors, singers, public speakers – acquire throat cancer. It's as if they are disappointed that their own words have so little meaning to the bigger world, while the words they are famous for speaking, hold so much more significance for so many.

The strength of the neck muscles denotes how high we can hold our head to face the world. Do we feel strong and confident as we look far ahead, or do we look downwards when walking?

As the neck is the division between the head and the body we can either integrate the two or keep them separate, which invariably leads us to disconnect the emotions as we begin to live in our heads, disregarding the needs of the body.

Words
The neck is very often where words get caught. They haven't come up far enough to be released through the mouth, but have become stuck as we talk of having "a frog in my throat"

or "got something caught in my throat." The words are almost there but are unable to be released, either because we don't want to offend or we are of fearful of the response. We clear the throat to be able to speak our intentions clearly, but who are we clearing it for, a boss, spouse, parents, or a group of people we wish to distance ourselves from? We also clear the throat when we feel nervous and say that we have a "frog in my throat" before speaking to groups.

Frogs are patient and and look as if they aren't paying attention, but as an insect passes they have the ability to snap it with their sticky tongue. The words we want to say may be stifled, but we should also be on our guard for suddenly lashing out and saying them at an inopportune moment. We may hit the bullseye, but then regret it! Frogs also croak and make unappealing noises—except to other frogs, one supposes—but, like butterflies, frogs symbolize new life as their eggs become little swimming tadpole which grow legs and then hop out of the water onto land where they can sit, catch flies and be content. So is the obstruction in our throat really a longing for a new life? And what words need to accompany a new life. "I'm leaving," perhaps? Leaving a relationship, marriage, job, location?

If the words are going in the opposite direction, from the mouth downwards, then we often have trouble "swallowing them." But words we are forced to swallow are usually indigestible and lead to digestive problems, much like undigested foods. If the food remains in the system too long, it becomes putrid, so is there a situation that is rotting from the inside out?

Getting anything caught in the throat, or any problem relating to the neck area, is usually connected to something distasteful. It won't go down, and it won't come back up, so sits in the middle deciding the best route to take. "Should I throw the remark back, or should I swallow my pride?" Words relating to the swallowing action, such as "I can't swallow this any longer," implies that someone is making us accept something distasteful. But who is it, a spouse, boss, someone in authority that we can't talk back to, a business partner who refuses to listen?

We ask kids who don't talk much or don't answer questions, if the "cat got your tongue," while never bothering to dig a little deeper to find out why they don't talk. Are they afraid of getting into trouble if they do speak? Afraid to tell the truth about something? Afraid of being bullied? Or feeling that no one is listening to them?

Sometimes we are wordless and let the actions speak for us as we tug on clothing that wraps around the throat, tug-

> John Gotti the Mafia Don, died of throat cancer while in jail. As a leading figure in the Mafia he was always the one to give the orders. In jail his voice was finally silenced.

ging to free the words. Many have attributed this action to having the umbilical cord wrapped around the neck during birth, and words that stick in the throat can produce the same action. We have a feeling of being slowly strangled and a longing to breathe freely. The tightening cuts off the passageway to free speech as it reduces the air flow. Waiting for the danger, either real or imaginary, to pass. Waiting for our turn to speak. Waiting for someone to listen.

We speak of others being "a pain in the neck," indicating that they have rigid thinking and won't see things our way, causing us to have a pain in our neck from the stress of the situation.

Rigid thinking also produces a stiff neck, which makes it difficult to turn the neck to see another point of view. If we have the pain, then what options do we have to satisfy both parties.

"Jumping down someone's throat," refer to words spoken too quickly and with too little thought, just as we "ram it down their throat" when we want to force an idea on others—forcing them to swallow it by force, not democratically. We can spit the words back if we so choose, but then we have to weigh that response too. Who will we be throwing the words back? What repercussions will it produce when the hastily spoken words can no longer be retracted. Things "stick in the throat" if we allow them, and then we often "cut our own throat" by not taking action, indicating that we are being self-destructive.

"A tickle in the throat" is just a small irritation that needs monitoring to make sure it doesn't become a full-blown cough, although a tickle can also imply something fun, so is it a good, or bad tickle? Nip the problem in the bud if it is negative. Otherwise, find out who is "tickling our fancy."
If asked to" cough it up" then we are to give up whatever is being asked for—money, information, other valuable things. It usually indicates that we don't have a choice but to obey, but if the one who must be obeyed is making us ill, then we need to find a way out of the situation. On the other hand, it may be a simple as coughing up the irritant so that we can move on. Once we really look at the event clearly, the decision may be ours, and not their, to make.

Doing something at "breakneck speed" is the same as driving fast and usually ends in a collision. Are we the ones going too fast, or are others? If we don't heed the warning, then we will probably finish "up to our neck" in something we don't want to be that far into. It may be a dangerous situation we are not able to extricate ourselves from, and will "get it in the neck" as we suffer the consequences. If a young person is speaking, listen to what they are really saying. Are they about to do something reckless, connected to driving or drugs, or something confrontational based on anger and irrational thinking?

"He's constantly sticking his neck out" we say of incautious people who leave themselves open to having their heads figuratively chopped off, as in business. Sometimes, though, reckless behavior can be good, as in taking a risk that may pay off, and people stick their necks out for good causes, political beliefs, and to fight for freedom of speech. Whistleblowers stick their necks out in the belief that the information should be known, even though it places them in danger, as the neck, once injured, can produce paralysis—as in job and economic loss—or even death.

Often, saying the words "I'm afraid to stick my neck out" implies that we want to stop the action before it starts, maybe because of a bully who constantly belittles us. Shrinking the neck down onto the shoulders gives the neck a little more protection from harm.

Feeling vindicated about someone who "got it in the neck" may make us feel better about a situation, but were they really at fault? We can say the words, but the body responds, and if we end up with neck pain then we need to see our part in the event. "Breathing down his neck" is a gentler form of wanting to hurt someone and implies the physical closeness of both parties: parent and child, boss and employee, or husband and wife. They are close enough to be able to breathe down the neck of the other to send a wordless message.

Those who say they are at the "end of my rope" are really in trouble emotionally and are probably very depressed. A rope around the neck, a noose, signifies the end, or the desire to put an end to whatever is troubling them. They are out of everything: money, energy, solutions, and now need external help.

See Lungs, Brain and Thyroid for additional information.

NOSE – Sinuses

Basic Anatomy

The nose is a protuberance in the central part of the face made from cartilage and bone, and, although many believe that it keeps growing throughout life, it actually stops growing after puberty. As we age we experience loss of muscle tone, bone and cartilage, causing the nose to droop a little, which tends to make it look bigger and longer.

Behind the nose is the nasal cavity, which extends back into the head and connects with the sinuses; a system of paired, hollow cavities in the skull—lined with a membrane—that sit behind the forehead, cheekbones and between the eye sockets. Sinusitis, a nasal congestion caused by an inflammation of the tissue, usually from bacteria or a virus, can create headaches around the eyes and forehead from the pressure buildup.

There are two passages in the nose called nasal cavities, divided by a partition called the septum, which opens into the nostrils. The nasal cavity filters the air we breath by removing dust particles, germs and other irritants and moistens the air to keep the airways from drying out.
These nasal cavities connect to the ear by way of the eustachian tubes, which run from the middle ear to the nose and throat. The eustachian tubes equalize pressure between the inner ear and the outside, which is why an infection occurs in the nose, ears and throat together.

The nose is also responsible for our sense of smell and taste, as the nerves signal information to the brain about what we are about to ingest. People who have trouble smelling usually have trouble tasting too.

Emotional disharmony

A sense of smell is a matter of safety and if this sense goes—often later in life—it can cause people to feel unsafe when alone or produce a fear of aging. Loss of smell is also connected to taste, which is connected to enjoyment of food and of life, so losing the sense of smell is like a loss of joy of who we were and what we might have accomplished. This loss may reflect a need to block out certain events, or a period of time, from our lives. Sometimes the sense of smell will return when we move into a better situation, which can be years after the initial loss.

Some smells are pleasant and evoke delightful memories, while others are unpleasant and recall the dentist, doctor, childhood visits to elderly relatives, rotting food, or other unpleasant situations. Distasteful smells also remind us of a particular person we may wish to forget. Pleasant smells, like perfumes, remind us of pleasurable times or lost loves.

Smells can represent nature and the outdoors, or indoor stuffiness, but if a stuffy nose happens only in certain indoor places and in certain company, then not only is the air a problem, but the people may also be toxic. If the difficulty occurs only at the workplace, then who or what event is causing the reaction? If breathing difficulties occur at home, then what room, or what person sets them off? We blame pets and other external factors for allergies and disregard the emotional content that is usually the trigger point. If the environment is stuffy, then where is the stuffiness coming from? Is it really an air quality problem, or something much more emotional?

The nose is connected to breathing, taking in air in order to live, so emotions around the nose connect to how we feel about being part of life and feeling that we have sufficient air to breathe. Childhood smells can be reassuring, such as odors of baking and foods that we liked; at other times they can dredge up bad memories such as alcohol and an alcoholic parent. Sometimes just one nostril closes or becomes smaller, obstructing the air we breathe, so is it the right or left one? Who or what are we blocking out and which side is the stronger one taking in the air?

Changing the shape of the nose with plastic surgery may make us feel better for a while, but if we don't also change the underlying emotions, then the original shape may return, especially if the reason for the surgery was to find a spouse, please others, or change our personality.

On the other hand, if the surgery is done to correct a breathing problem, and the cause of the blockage is really a spouse, partner or coworker causing a stifling environment, then the problem will return—unless the emotions are also cleared. Very often we focus on the medical problem but not the emotional one.

Most men don't seem to have a problem with their nose size—possibly because they believe the old adage that nose size correlates with penis size—while most women want a small, upturned nose to make them look more attractive. And they may be right, as a naturally upturned nose seems to suggest a more cheerful disposition.

The dissatisfaction with the size and shape is probably due to the fact that it is in the central part of the face. The eyes and mouth are located around the nose, but the nose is the central external object and so has a very big emotional impact on how we interact with others and how we view ourselves, both from the front and the side. If one side of the face is more attractive than the other, which side is it, the analytical right side or the more creative left side? The muscles of the face also connect to the muscles in the neck and shoulders, so there could be a distortion of the muscles on one side of the face, rather than nose size being the problem.

Snoring, which is associated with stress, occurs during sleep and is related to the passage of air through the nostrils. Men tend to snore more than women, but women are also more likely to deal with stress in words, while men find other outlets. Snoring reflects fear and apprehension without words, as the nose and mouth cavities of the nose deny enough air into the lungs. What obstructions happen during the day that block the airwaves at night.? Who or what is causing the delay in getting air into the passages, someone in business, or a social, or family situation?

Colds block the air passages, making us blow the nose repeatedly in order to clear them, and a streaming nose shows a desire to cry and release pent-up emotions. We may want time out to grieve for some past situation, or for ourselves. Multiple colds per year, every year, reflects an emotional problem that keeps recurring and is never released, maybe the response to the death of a loved one, the loss of innocence in childhood, a childhood lost due to taking care of a sick parent, or the loss of a past relationship. If a particular time of year, or a certain date or situation produces a cold, then look at what prompted it. Adults make the excuse that they catch colds from their kids in school, but healthy people with a strong immune system can ward off colds, so the weakness is caused by something else.

Constant sinus troubles are a reminder that the problem isn't draining away as it should, and so mucus is building up, along with the bacteria and irritants that are not able to be released. Bacteria that is allowed to fester usually lead to a full-blown illness. What is being allowed to build up, resentment, anger, fear? And who or what is causing the buildup? A situation that was never fully resolved? A death that was never fully accepted, and the unfinished grieving has now become a long term sinus problem? Tears that were never released when they should have been because of wanting to appear strong? A fear of releasing the tears and what it will bring up?

Words

In the West, words about noses are often derogatory, which may be a big reason why people are dissatisfied with their nose size in the first place. The nose is something we poke into things we shouldn't be poking into: we use the term "nosey parkers" to describe intrusive people, and we tell them to "keep your nose out of my business" and stop meddling. We tell others to "keep your nose to the grindstone" to make them work harder and "look down our nose" at those less fortunate, and "lead them by the nose" when we think they are weak and naive.

We make others "pay through the nose" if we think we can get away with it, and then delight in their irritation as we put their "nose out of joint" and "rub their nose in it" as a reminder—which we also do to toilet train dogs! We don't actually want to hit them—in case they hit us back—but we do want to send them a strong message to back off. Taking delight in another's downfall indicates our own lack of power, so what are we being forced to accept that we'd rather not? What are we trying to make up for? Someone who humiliated us, someone who removed our ability to have power over our own life and left us with a "bad smell" about the entire situation? Or are we on the receiving end, feeling powerless to stop the humiliating action, that like a "slow drip," won't turn off?

Constantly "feeling stuffed up" is to have stale air surrounding us, maybe coming from someone who is stuffy and self-serving, not allowing us to breathe freely as they slowly suffocate us, our ideas, our projects, and "take the wind out of our sails." Is a situation stifling our creativity, or others who will not allow us to be part of a project? Someone who always puts down our efforts? A relationship where not enough air is allowed to flow between us and a spouse, parent, coworker, boss, partner? When we can't breathe freely, we gasp for air as the oxygen needed for life has become blocked, but often we are the ones who block our own way because of our own insecurity, or sense of being unworthy.

> Jimmy Durante, nicknamed The Schnoz, was a comedian and singer in the 1940's. His nose was insured for $50,000. In that same period an average income for the year was $2,000.

We can also refer to feeling stuffed up, as in being obese or being congested in other parts of the body, such as the stomach or colon. "Stuff" is not moving through the way it should, or not moving through with ease, whether it's in the body, home, or office. We collect "stuff" in our homes that often prevents us from being social and inviting others into our space, and emotions that are "stuffed" together can lead to physical or emotional illness.

In some cultures, a large nose is considered an asset, even something to feel proud of. We use the term "nosed forward" or "won by a nose" when someone wins a race, whether in

The Body's Emotional Imprint

business or physically, while others "arrive right on the nose" and are punctual, which is a quality to admire. In this context the nose implies success, especially if we can "smell trouble" or "smell success."

When we "smell a rat," we don't trust others or our ability to deal with them, and if we are taken advantage of and "didn't smell a rat" until it was too late, we may be angry with ourselves for allowing it to happen. In that case the nose failed to warn us soon enough, and may cause us to disregard other danger signs, too, such as smoke—signifying things about to erupt in our life—or the "smell" from a rotting relationship that needs attention.

Some make a living by their nose, as they smell wines, perfumes and foods in order to make their product more attractive to their customers. New cars smell of leather to induce us to buy the smell, rather than the car. When a smell is unacceptable, we conceal it with one that is acceptable, like a room freshener. It doesn't eliminate the underlying odor, but it does conceal it. We do the same thing when we hide problems instead of addressing them.

The way we view the nose, as an asset or something detrimental, usually correlates with how clear our breathing is—and how clear-thinking we are. When we "take our fill of air" we feel good about taking our share without guilt, but breathing problems suggest that we are not sure about how much we are allowed and whether we have the right to take it.

See Lungs and Chest for additional information.

OVARIES – Uterus

Basic Anatomy

The uterus, shaped a little like a hollow inverted triangle the size of a small pear, lies inside the pelvic bone and functions for reproductive purposes only. Protruding into the vagina at the narrow end and into the abdominal cavity at the other, it tilts forward over the bladder.

The ovaries, small almond-shaped organs about the size of a grape and measuring about an inch in length after puberty, are held by several connective ligaments that branch out one each side of the top of the uterus. Part of the menstruation process, which starts around the age of 13, the ovaries in a female fetus are usually formed by the third month of pregnancy. At birth the ovaries contain 1 – 2 million eggs, but by puberty have dwindled down to around 300,000 immature eggs—although only about 500 hundred of them will ever be released, at the rate of one single egg each month. At menopause, the ovaries shrink and stop releasing eggs.

The pituitary gland, situated at the base of the brain, controls the ovaries by way of messages from the hypothalamus, the link between the nervous system and the endocrine system, and is responsible for maintaining the body's internal balance, known as homeostasis. The hormones progesterone and estrogen are produced and released by the ovaries and are necessary for normal reproductive function.

Emotional disharmony

The reproductive system—menstruation to menopause— relates to how women feel about their role in society as mothers, caretakers and career women. Menstruation problems, such as bloating, swelling of breasts, PMS, infertility problems, menopause, cancer and other conditions, all link to how women feel about the entire process of being female, from birth to death and all the stages between—body image, sexuality, motherhood, and aging.

Throughout the ages the female body has been promoted to that of a goddess, reduced to that of a whore, and has touched on everything in between, so it comes as no surprise that women today are taught to devalue their worth on the one hand, and think of themselves as superwomen, on the other. But trying to be all the images is taking its toll, especially as many men want a bad girl in the bedroom, but a good girl to marry!

The color red is the color of blood and of life as it pulses through the body. Unfortunately, menstruation, is also linked to the color red, blood and pain. If we damage the skin and it bleeds, pain usually follows, and menstruation is seen by many as something unpleasant and to be feared, both by women who experience it, and men who don't understand it.

The media constantly focus on the negative side of menstruation—it sells an assortment of products—but they don't report on the positive side, which for some women is a time of high energy, a time to be creative, a time of doing, a time of clarity, and seeing it as a gift rather than something to fear. For them, womanhood is a celebration.

The reproductive system also represents women standing up for who they are—as protectors, nurturers and caretakers— of both the past generation and the future one. The way women feel about the role can class them as either warriors or worn down. The delicate balancing act of juggling family, career and personal needs, is difficult, but if there is a hormonal balance, then all the emotions will be unbalanced, too.

Bloating signifies a blowing up, in this case the breasts, but it can also refer to a problem that has blown up due to inequality, perhaps related to a job where being female means being paid less than the men, or given greater responsibility without the perks. A humiliating situation that reminds us each month as the bloating appears, that it's time to face the inequality and deal with it, either by leaving or speaking up about it. Men ogling the breasts at that time of the month is another reminder of the power men have over women in the work place—unless the table is turned and the woman takes advantage of looking sexy.

Menstrual cramps—painful spasmodic muscular contractions—are the bottling up of emotions as the blockage forces the body to double over in pain and into the fetal position, just as it was before the pain of childbirth released us as newborns. A desire to go within and back to the source where we were safe, away from the pain of being an adult in an adult world. What do we really want to say but cannot now that we are an adult? What emotions are we bottling up? What responsibilities do we have that we need to release? And who or what is the pain connected to?

Fertility and uterine problems relate to how we accept motherhood. Are we receiving mixed messages about having children? Are we ready to have them, or is someone pushing us, such as parents and in-laws? Are we afraid to give birth? Afraid of the pain and the responsibility?

Pregnancy, for some, is a form of control, a way to take charge of the one thing they can control—the act of giving birth. It can be control over parents and in-laws who want to be grandparents, or of husbands and partners who want to father a child—think Henry VIII who desperately wanted a son! Problems with a pregnancy or birth can often be traced back to how we felt about being a mother at the time of conception. Did we want to get pregnant or just have fun? Were we coerced into having sex or did we do it willingly? Or was it an obligation from some past event—dinner bought, money loaned, a deal?

Ovaries are the starting place for the eggs awaiting their turn to be transform into a new life. The way we view our own life and the lives of others is linked to how we feel about our eggs. Do they represent something to be disposed of, or something to be care for? Do we value them, and ourselves, or do we want the process to be over as soon as possible? Ovarian cysts are a wake-up call about how we feel about being a mother and how we view our relationship to a new life, or to our own new life. A cyst is something small that grows, often filled with fluid but sometimes solid, so what emotions are contained in that growth? Fluid as in tears, or something rock hard that we will not give in to? Do we have a partner to raise babies with? Do we want one, or are we ambivalent? Is our mate a willing father-to-be, or is there resistant? Do we want to be a single mother, or do we need a partner to give us love and support? A growth usually makes the process of reproduction difficult, so where is the resistance taking place?

Menopause is the end of the monthly cycles, signifying freedom for many who have children and others who have no interest in having them, and disappointment for those who want children. In this society menopause has also come to mean the end of sexual attraction, of being needed and wanted, and of being useful. Women have been browbeaten into believing that this is the end of anything creative—many see the act of giving birth as creative—and that there is nothing much to look forward to after menopause, instead of seeing it as the opening up of something new, exciting and burden-free.

Menopause often produces hot flashes, during which heat washes across the face, upper body, or the entire body, and produces sweating and rapid heart beat—much like great sex. Unfortunately, we connect sweating to nervousness and heat to burning and scarring—in this case, seeing the future and usefulness of women going up in smoke. If we held the image of sweat, heat and rapid heartbeat connected to a power surge and great sex, then maybe menopause would represent the dissolving of the old and the beginning of something new.

For some, menopause does represent freedom, freedom from fear of an unintended pregnancy. Freedom to say anything. Freedom from the restrictions of society. Freedom to dance, sing, laugh, or be grouchy, cantankerous and even a crone.

A hysterectomy is an operation to remove the uterus—partially or totally—and is usually performed on older women, although it can be performed at any age. Many hysterectomies are unnecessary and are really performed to replace the feeling of being unloved. Perhaps the marriage has become unfulfilling? The children are grown and have left home, and now there is little reason to hold the marriage together. Or the husband is unfaithful, leaving the wife to feel unimportant and unwanted. The uterus is about childbirth and life, and its removal signifies the end of that ability. Or it can be a way not to have children, and for some, can signify a release from pain, allowing freedom from all that it stands for.

Health problems associated with the ovaries and uterus are a reflection of who women are today and the stress and mixed message they receive about being female in a male-dominated society. Goddess or whore. Mother or career woman. Supermom or failure. Problems in this area come from the conflict of juggling a home, a job, spouse, children, elderly parents, and finding time to be fulfilled oneself.

Words

For many women, the reproductive part of the body has negative connotations, and the words referring to it are often ones of putting trust in specialists, instead of the natural ability of women to know their own bodies. Women often accept the words of others—usually men—who are considered specialists in the areas of childbirth, raising children, menstruation and menopause.

Women especially, tend to talk negatively about their monthly periods, saying, "I've got the curse," as if a higher, or perhaps a lower, power really did have a hand in it. This time of the month is also referred to as "being on the rag," which comes from the fact that women would cut up pieces of cloth, called rags, before pads and tampons were invented. According to some interpretations, the term "ragtime" music refers to this sense of the word rag: in brothels, prostitutes who and had their monthly periods had to sing and entertain the customers instead of having sex. It was a way to keep the customers happy and remaining in the brothels.

Perhaps if we saw it as a "something to sing about" instead of something to dread, then there would be fewer psychological problems connected to menstruation.

Talking about "that time of the month" as if it is something to be feared, and believing that "all women have period pain/bloating" as a natural course of events—which it isn't—and accepting without question that hot flashes come with menopause, and that nausea comes with pregnancy, really reflects the brainwashing that is imposed on women, believing that their natural bodily functions must be both painful and debilitating.

Blood, in many cultures, represents life and the color red is considered vital, which is why brides wear red. Western culture sees blood representing the end of life as it drains away, instead of the renewal that it could be.

Hysterectomies are the second most frequently performed surgical procedure in the U.S. for women -- after cesarean section -- and between 85% to 90% of them are unnecessary. It's a multibillion dollar industry.

Even though most women don't think too much about their uterus, it does symbolize growth, either on a personal level or in terms of things we actively do: appearance, work, family, and so the sentences we say often start with "I'm not good at......." as we devalue ourselves and our abilities, of not being a good mother, not sure about having children, afraid of taking charge of our own body or career.

The words often reflect our chosen profession or job, and how qualified we feel doing the work. Are we insecure, or are we ambitious? Do we say "I know what I want to do in life and I'm going for it," or " I think having children would

The Body's Emotional Imprint

impede my progress?" Is the word "child" the focal word, or are words connected to the job more central? The way we phrase sentences indicates what our main worry/focus is. If we find ourselves saying "I"m not sure this is the right time to have kids," then we are ambivalent about career and mothering, but saying "I need to work on my career before I have kids" indicates that the focus is on the career.

"I feel so flushed" for many menopausal women means they see heat as an embarrassment instead of a power surge, but in the game of poker having "a royal flush" is a good thing. The game is won, just as it is for many menopausal women, and a new game is beginning.

See Heart, Chest and Neck for additional information.

PANCREAS – Diabetes

Basic Anatomy

The pancreas is a dual-purpose gland that produces several important hormones for the blood and also enzymes to assist in the digestive process. A long, tapered organ about 6 inches long, it lies behind the stomach and extends from the right side with most of it over to the left side of the body. The head—the wide part of the pancreas on the right side—is connected to the small intestine by way of the duodenum, which is the first part of the small intestines that begins the absorption of nutrients from partially digested foods. If the ducts leading from the pancreas become blocked, then digestive fluids build up, producing acute pancreatitus—severe inflammation.

The pancreas produces pancreatic fluid called insulin, a hormone that helps transfer glucose into the cells of the body, and into the liver where it is stored as glycogen. Pancreatic juices also contain digestive enzymes that help to break down carbohydrates, proteins, fats and acids. Some cells also secretes bicarbonate, which neutralizes stomach acids.

If the pancreas fails to produce enough insulin, then diabetes occurs. Diabetes is a disease in which the blood sugar levels are too high. The hormone Insulin is necessary to transport glucose into the cells, which then enables the body to utilize it as energy. Although most pancreatic activity goes into the digestive process, it is the insulin activity that usually produces problems.

Type 1 diabetes occurs when the body produces little or no insulin to handle the amount of glucose in the body and so requires insulin—usually in the form of injections—to help the body utilize glucose appropriately. The disease usually appears in childhood.

Type 2 diabetes is much more common and usually affects adults who may be able to produce some insulin but can't utilize it effectively—called insulin resistance. When people are insulin resistant, glucose builds up in the blood instead of being absorbed by the cells. Diet and exercise can play their part in managing and preventing it.

Hypoglycemia occurs when there is not enough sugar in the blood, or there is too much insulin, causing weakness and dizziness. Diabetics may have this too if the insulin intake isn't balanced against the food intake and exercise exertion.

Cancer of the pancreas can be felt as pain in the upper abdomen, or loss of appetite, weight loss, and jaundice if the head of the pancreas obstructs the bile duct. The cancer forms when cells grow uncontrollably rather than developing into healthy, normal tissue, and as these abnormal cells continue to divide and multiply, they form into tumors to interfere with the main pancreatic process.

Emotional disharmony

The pancreas pertains to both the giving and receiving of sweetness, and so cancer and diabetes are indicative of sweetness not being reciprocated or of not allowing ourselves to accept sweetness when it is offered. A large percentage of our foods and drinks now have some form of sweetness added to them—usually artificial—and feeling unloved, we often consume sugary things as a replacement for what is missing emotionally.

The pancreas also breaks down proteins, carbohydrates and fats, and we may feel incapable of breaking out of the life we are living, or unable to use the resources presented to us because of others—or we ourselves, through fear and insecurity are blocking the way.

Usually, the body regulates how sugar is utilized, but not letting in enough sweetness for our needs, leads the body to compensates by either being overly sweet or left unable to utilize the glucose in a way that will give us energy to do the things we wish to do, taking away the joys of life.
Diabetes was a disease of older people, but now many more children are being diagnosed with it, indicating that there is something missing from their lives when it comes to love and attention, or lack of attention from busy working parents. It's a sad commentary on society and how unconnected people feel.

Once a year, on Valentine's Day, we give chocolates as a way to show love to another and we give them to people who are recovering from illness to show we care. The more expensive the chocolates, the more it equates with the level of care we wish to show, which is why chocolate is a good mood food.

Diabetes is a disease of the blood, and blood circulates around the body freely giving out oxygen and nutrients to the entire system. People with Type 2 diabetes, which is the most common form, hoard sugar so that they don't feel deprived. If others won't love them and give them the affection they need, then they will love themselves by storing their own sweetness.

Emotionally, people with diabetes are often those who have a difficult time with relationships and with knowing how much of themselves to give and how much to hold back. They struggle to find the emotional boundaries between giving and receiving. They can also feel smothered with superficial affection from family members, perhaps an aging parent or needy siblings, who are actually manipulating the situation to fulfill their own needs, and who cling for support, draining all the sweetness to themselves.

We eat sweet and fattening foods for comfort when we are feeling depressed or deprived, but filling up with chips, cookies, pastries and chocolate bars is an indication of how lonely and unconnected we really feel. Glucose provides energy, so if energy levels are low and we need a chocolate bar in the middle of the afternoon to keep going, then it may be connected to where we work or the type of work we do. Do we feel supported or do we feel that we are giving while others take advantage of our generosity? Is there a lot of give and take in the workplace where the workload is shared, or is it one-side?

Chocolate may be a quick fix for a time, but it does nothing for the long-term problem. Those who are depleted of energy during the day are often on diets, cutting out carbohydrates in order to lose weight, but then sabotage themselves by eating sugary snacks in order to fill that void. As the guilt increases, so do the cravings for more sugar and fatty snacks, which brings up all the negative emotions of feeling weak-willed, disgusted and full of self-loathing—all the reason many feel they are unlovable in the first place

Hypoglycemia occurs when there is not enough sugar in the bloodstream; it causes weakness and dizziness. As children we wait for love to come from our parents, and usually it does, but if the parents seem uncaring then we will feel deprived. Often the origins of our neediness come from a childhood where we saw love and attention go to others, or had parents, who themselves, grew up with little love and are now incapable giving it to others. Or we may block love from getting to us and fear getting involved with anyone who we believe will fall short of our expectations. Children who were hurt or who never knew the kind of love they craved, were usually told that it's selfish to attend to their own needs and not the needs of others, preventing them from knowing they deserve to be loved and that it's all right to ask for it.

We need glucose to keep our cells functioning well and to keep them balanced in order to maintain good health. Without the ability to distribute the sugars, we will become either deprived or overloaded, and in life, too, we need to be able to balance things: work, family, relationships. If work becomes more important than family, then there is an imbalance that will make family members also feel deprived, and sweetness that is blocked can turn into sourness, producing ill feelings.

Taking from life what we need is a form of self-love, which, if blocked turns to anger and resentment against ourselves. Daily injections, required by diabetics, are a constant reminder to allow more affection in, or have it pumped into the body by some other means. Some learn the lesson and move away from the daily grind; others do not.

Pancreatic cancer is a growing of the barrier that blocks the relationships we most crave, those with parents, spouse or offspring. It's also forgiveness and letting go of the sourness and resentment that have allowed the cancerous cells to multiply. We are often afraid to show our more disagreeable side to the outside world, preferring to show a nicer, more cloying side, while carrying the anger internally, which then becomes

The Body's Emotional Imprint

a diseased organ. Or our resentment will often manifest as control, of the emotions both at work and with the family, as the dominant side crushes the softer side that is hurting.

The disease is also about carrying the hurt around for a very long time, with the sorrow and sadness that goes with it. A hurt that was never released and has now grown so big that it is devouring us.

Words

Words that reflect love and being needed are often connected to the pancreas. Words that show a need to be needed, a need for acceptance, which we often push away at the same time. "Now that my children are grown, they no longer need me" shows the recognition that we no longer feel wanted and that the love is being passed on to others: a spouse, a child or a partner. Our role has decreased, theirs has increased. It can also be that we no longer want to accept the affection as it may force us to forgive a past action that we would rather not release. Accepting warmth from others may indicate weakness or neediness, and as children, we may have formed a barrier in order to give the appearance of strength, while the hurt was buried.

Hiding a hurt within the body, will at some point, resurface, just as dead bodies in the attic usually do—and just like dead bodies it will return in a festering state.

When we no longer feel agreeable, we feel hostile towards others. Or we call someone a "sour puss" when they show no positive emotions to others. Anything sour causes the mouth to pucker up and not allow anything in. We sense sourness by taste and words, and often it comes from a life of hardship and the feeling that others have had it easy and somehow never "paid their dues." Elderly people who are ill-tempered and disagreeable are often thought of as bitter and unlovable, when in truth they may be hiding their sense of hopelessness, or an illness.

Energy is connected to glucose and all things sweet. We eat a chocolate bar when we need a quick fix during the day as we say, "I've lost all my energy." But it could be that we are eating the wrong foods to give us long-lasting energy, or that we are in a job that is boring and no longer challenging, and no longer motivates us to do much. We are not "loving the work" and are just marking time. How much of diabetes is related to feeling that life has little to offer and that there is no way out of a dead-end job, marriage, or lifestyle.

In the outer world, too, we are also beginning to lack conventional fuels for energy and are now resorting to new ones that require an overuse of water and chemicals and the destruction of the earth. So a lack of personal energy is also a fear about our future with regard to jobs, health and the implosion of a once-abundant planet.

Women say, "He used to be sweet on me" about a relationship that is no longer fulfilling as the love has moved on. But who stopped the love? Often the one with pancreatic problems is the one who is no longer willing to balance the relationship and has become too needy for the partner to respond to. Or, maybe the pancreatic problem has made it difficult to be attentive to their partner, and ill health has overridden the ability to care.

We use the word "sweet" and "honey" to show affection for family members, and calling someone a "sweetie" describes someone good and pleasurable who feeds our needs. But the term can also be used in a derogatory way when said to someone of lower class or position, usually at work or in social situations. It can also be used to make others feel subordinate.

Sweetness is also sticky and cloying, and stickiness is difficult to get off as it leaves marks on things, just as sticky sentiment can be overwhelming and excessive. Clingy people have to be disconnected or "washed out" before they leave too many "marks" that are difficult to clean off, and usually the only way to disconnect them is to display coldness and indifference.

Steve Jobs of Apple fame, died from pancreatic cancer at the age of 56. We think of the rich and famous living perfect lives, but like the rest of us, they too, carry emotional scars. It's difficult to feel self-love if you're put up for adoption and booted out of your own business.

Too much sweetness can also make us feel sluggish and tired. We experience a quick high, then a crash, as we complain, "I just can't seem to get going this morning." Morning is often the time when we skip a meal, leaving us to grab something sugary to eat on the way to work, a quick sugar fix that quickly subsides so that we need another quick sugary fix midmorning.

Sometimes we are unable to hang onto the warm feeling of a situation, as it is flushed through the system too quickly, causing us to feel resentment at not having had the time for a loving relationship. Unable to balance the love with other things we wish to do in the belief that we have to give up one in order to have the other. This feeling often comes from growing up in a family that could never find a balance, a family unable to give love, or that withheld it, or used love as a form of control. Often, the compensation for lack of attention and time comes in the form of sugary rewards, a junk food outing, or rewards of money and gifts, which somehow are never given freely. Many adults remember that "mother/father always had to have control." Substituting gifts for the affectionate relationships that most children crave, will turn them into sugar-eating adults with few boundaries, who try to capture love any way they can.

See the Liver, Small Intestine and Obesity for additional information.

PINEAL GLAND

Basic Anatomy

Situated in the mid-brain between the two hemispheres, the pineal gland is a reddish color about the size of a grain of rice, and is part of the endocrine system (hormone secreting glands). It releases a substance into the bloodstream called melatonin, which regulates the biological sleep cycle, and serotonin, also known as 5-hydroxytryptamine (5-HT). Serotonin acts as a neurotransmitter, relaying messages from one area of the brain to another, and although it is manufactured in the brain, 90% of it is found in the digestive tract and in blood platelets.

Light exposure that penetrates the eyes' retina has an indirect link to the pineal gland via the hypothalamus, and balancing darkness with daylight is part of the process that enables good health and an ability to function well when awake, as well as to sleep soundly through the night. Sunshine also affects the brain, which decreases production of melatonin during the day and increases that of serotonin when exposed to the sun.

A lack of sunlight, often caused by seasonal variations, can produce mood disorders such as depression and sleep depravation, which, in turn, produce varying levels of melatonin, leading to tiredness and an unbalanced sleep cycle.

The pineal gland is larger in very young children and shrinks after the age of about seven years. It may influence sexual development, which could account for the irregular sleep cycles and behavioral problems in teenagers.

Emotional disharmony

Like many areas in life, small things can often have the biggest effect and the pineal gland is no exception. It has been called the "seat of the soul" and the "third eye," but its main function is to make the hormone melatonin, which may regulate the onset of puberty. The gland lies buried in the mid brain at the base of the corpus callosum, the nerve bundles that connect the left and right hemispheres of the brain, so balance in all things is important, especially the ability to see both sides of an issue.

Before women embarked on careers and were supposed to stay home as "happy homemakers," they often went to the doctor complaining of not feeling well generally. The doctor, finding no real illness after a thorough checkup, usually told them that the illness was all in their heads. Now we know that the diagnosis was probably correct. To the doctor it was an imaginary illness; to the woman it was an unfulfilled spiritual yearning coupled with lack of outside contact and sunlight.

Very little research has been collected on the pineal gland, except to connect it to our circadian rhythms and reproductive hormones, but as we know so little about the gland, it is probably premature to disregard it as of little importance to our emotional makeup.

Before the 1960's, women were not allowed the freedom to think for themselves, and many never questioned their position. They ruled the home, but not the money, and men worked—and controlled the money. To the doctors of the day, many of the illnesses women complained of were presumed to be psychosomatic. In truth, they were probably connected to the pineal gland, and the real illness was boredom and not being allowed to participate in a closed society.

The inability to use intellectual potential will eventually produce frustration, hopelessness and illness of the body and the mind.

Women, who are much more intuitive than men and often know and see the truth about a society, were not able to voice their opinions, especially in public where they were supposed to be polite and acquiesce to men, were left feeling frustrated—which is where Sigmund Freud enters. Considered the founding father of psychoanalysis, Freud opposed women's emancipation and believed they were dominated by their reproductive function. He also acknowledged that after thirty years of research, he still didn't know what women wanted! How much of illness today is from unhappy, unfulfilled and incomplete lives—and from working in dead end jobs?

As light, and especially sunlight, is so important to our health, so a regular sleep cycle is also important. The pineal gland responds to the natural flow of daytime into nighttime, and our biological clocks are timed to specific hours of the 24-hour cycle, with peaks and valleys occurring throughout that time. Some of us are night people and some work better in the morning, but trying to change the cycle is difficult. When sleep patterns are interrupted, irritability and fatigue set in, and it is often lack of light that produces depression and food cravings. So how much of being overweight is connected to lack of daylight, especially as many of us in the West work 9-5 jobs where in winter, we get up in the dark, come home in the dark, and work indoors under fluorescent lights during the daylight hours.

Sleeping well is imperative to our health, but in our culture very few people wake up refreshed, and that may be partly due to electronics that take up our time at night. But if the sleep pattern is constantly interrupted, there may be a deeper reason, one that goes back to childhood. Perhaps it was an alcoholic father who always came home late and then became abusive, or one who abused his children, sexually or physically, making it impossible for them to relax and sleep well. We don't sleep well when we are stressed and fearful, or when there is a situation that needs attention, or a nagging problem that needs finality. There may even be a much deeper emotional problem that needs to be recognized, one related to a fear of death or suffocation.

The pineal gland contains the highest concentration of fluoride in the body, and calcification of the pineal gland is usually connected to aging, but it seems that it can also be caused by the accumulated amounts of sodium fluoride which attach magnetically to the gland to form calcium phosphate crystals. Some research also seems to indicate that this may be a reason why girls menstruate much earlier than previous generations and a reason why we have IQ and memory problems. As we now add fluoride to much of our water supply, maybe we should spend more money on researching this question and less on pushing fluoride into communities.

Words

Often we don't have words to express how we feel or where a problem lies, all we do know is that something "feels off" or that it is too difficult to "get at." There is a feeling of worry, a disconnect, an unnamed fear somewhere in the head that has no words to describe it.

When we speak of a problem being "in my head" or of "knowing something intuitively," we think of women speaking, while men have "gut reactions" and talk of "knowing" something. As the pineal gland is in the middle of the head, it suggests that men and women have a different interpretation on how we react to situations: women believe they know, men know they know—even though the knowing may be wrong! This may be the reason why women's intuition isn't taken seriously, while men's gut reaction is—and why we have an imbalance between the two.

When we feel well rested and "lighthearted" we enjoy life, feel excited about the future and put plans into motion to start a new venture, business or baby. Or we "put plans into action" for projects we wish to move along. We want to "grow" in esteem at work and to be taken seriously for our efforts. These are all words that pertain to "moving up" in the world and feeling good about life, and if problems do arise then we "sleep on it" in order to find a solution, knowing that one will be found.

> Called the "Third Eye" by many, Rene Descartes regarded the pineal gland as the seat of the soul and the place where thoughts are formed.

Sometimes we are so overjoyed that we feel "giddy and light-headed," but it can also imply that we lack balance. People who have "sunny" dispositions are usually fun to be around and are the optimists and problem solvers, while those who feel the opposite are "dark" and "gloomy" and lack light in their lives, which probably comes from a lack of sunshine and Vitamin D. We naturally want to "grow towards the light" just as vegetation does, and as the body cannot make Vitamin D, the main source of it comes from the sun as the skin absorbs it.

Feeling the need to "go outdoors" or "get some fresh air" is often a sign that we are in need of more natural light.

Fluorescent light drains the energy of both the body and the brain and can make us feel "lightheaded" as we lose our concentration. This can affect kids as they sit under fluorescent light for most of the school day—at the same time that they are experiencing puberty. So could the problem with unruly teens and those with learning problems be connected to the lack of natural light, especially sunshine, which is a full-spectrum light—one that includes the range of wavelengths necessary to sustain life on Earth?

As it drains energy from the body, fluorescent light can give the skin a grayish pallor and can also trigger headaches, fatigue, anxiety and irritability, feelings that we associate with some sleep disorders. Lack of sleep can make us feel grumpy and can also cause us to "snap" at others or lead us to feel "unbalanced" as the day-to-night cycle is disrupted.

Irritation can also come from a calcified pineal gland, or even a kidney stone, as the friction tends to "rub people" the wrong way, which in relationships can cause discord as the conflict escalates. Hard things rubbing against soft objects can cause friction which is detrimental to our ability to move forward, and may force others to abandon their relationship with us as the conflict escalates.

How we feel internally usually translates outwards to how we treat others. If we have balance in our lives, then we are much more likely to treat others with fairness.

See Kidney, Brain, Skin and Pituitary for additional information.

PITUITARY GLAND

Basic Anatomy

The pituitary gland is the size of a pea and sits in a small, bony cavity at the base of the brain, behind the bridge of the nose and between the eyes, where the optic nerves carry information from the eyes to the back of the brain. The pituitary is often called the master gland since it controls most of the other endocrine glands—the network of glands that secrete hormones directly into the blood stream. It is regulated by a region in the brain called the hypothalamus, which is situated just above the pituitary and links the nervous system to the other glands via the pituitary.

The gland secretes hormones that are essential for normal growth and height development during childhood and adolescence, and for cell reproduction and regeneration. The secreted hormones are also responsible for sexual growth enabling puberty, fertility and pregnancy, as they regulate testosterone and promote sperm production in men, and regulate estrogen and stimulate ovulation and the production of milk in the mammary glands in women. The pituitary also orchestrates the secretion of hormones from other glands: from the thyroid to regulate metabolism, from the nervous system to regulate growth, and from the adrenals to stimulate the production of cortisol.

The gland has two parts, the anterior and the posterior lobes, each of which releases different hormones that affect bone growth and other gland activity. The anterior lobe produces hormones that affect the adrenals, ovaries and testes, while the posterior lobe affects the absorption of water into the kidneys. In adults the latter is also important for maintaining muscle and bone mass.

Dwarfism, gigantism and stunted growth occur occasionally, and link to too much or too little growth hormone, although, malnutrition and random genetic mutation, of either the sperm or the egg, are a more likely cause of the conditions.

Emotional disharmony

When we think of a master, we tend to think of someone who is all-knowing and possesses information that others don't, someone who gives directions and is given deferential treatment, and one who shows great proficiency in a chosen field.

If the master gland isn't functioning well, then it can't give directions to the other glands, meaning it isn't delegating well. The head is considered the thinking area, the master of the body, the place where messages are processed and then delivered. How well we delegate in situations where we are expected to take charge, will show in how strong and healthy we feel. Do we possess that mastery, or are we the one who sits back and waits for others to move forward and take control—and then silently resent every minute of it?

Organs work in their own areas: the heart pumps life into us, the liver is the sorting office, the kidneys keep the water works flowing, and the glands are the busybodies who work all over the place. And as the endocrines secrete hormones into the blood stream, the emotions are connected to the body's pulsating blood flow, which if blocked, or pumping too forcefully will create problems both physically and emotionally. Feeling pressure at work or at home can cause the glands to overreact, especially the adrenal and thyroid glands, and produce a constant level of stress, which, if not treated, will create an imbalance throughout the entire system as the hormones careen out of control.

The pituitary is necessary for the stability of our emotional well-being, and it can also cause us to feel moody and out of sorts without quite knowing why. Growth in one part of our lives can often cause an imbalance in another, whether it's starting a baby or a business, or changing direction, especially if the growth is unwanted or forced upon us. An imbalance in hormonal activity can make us feel off balance, too, as if the ground is shifting beneath our feet and we are unable to stand firmly, leaving us unable to take a stand for what we want and believe.

If we don't feel grounded and secure, whether at work, home or in relationships, then we feel disconnected from others, and since the pituitary gland is so important to our growth cycle, a problem here could be traced back to a sexual problem in our childhood or teen years. Any hormones interrupted at that point, either from illness, parental control, or sexual abuse, will become unbalanced in later life. The teenage years are very traumatic for many, and often what happens during those years stays with us forever, unless we are able to disconnect the words and images in question.

Connected to our development, and especially to the female element of procreation, the endocrine system is linked to the things we hope to create: a new business, relationship, marriage, or a change of profession or location. We have to feel strong enough emotionally to deal with the ups and downs that come with the creating, otherwise, we will be on a roller coaster that can leave us feeling exhausted, despondent and apathetic.

Growing a business, project, or family is much easier if it is done slowly and with thought, rather than built on speed, when it might grow too quickly for us to handle. It requires much less effort to reach our full potential—and hit great heights—when we take the time to think about what we really want to achieve before we set off on the journey. This also applies to weight loss and doing crash diets, which take the weight off fast, but then put the weight back on just as quickly.

Words

Anything linked to growth is usually positive, as it reflects optimism, but things can also grow out of control if left unattended. Feeling that things are "out of control" can pertain to life, health, relationships, a business or project, and may also relate to an impending trip or marriage whose preparations are spiraling out of control. Or we may know someone with an addiction who is out of control, or even ourselves, and refuse to acknowledge it. Fires burn out of control, taking everything with them, so if we feel that things are running too fast and too hot, then we, or they, need outside intervention.

Relinquishing control to another usually leads to a complete breakdown in a relationship, with a spouse, business partnership, or boss, or a project or event that becomes unworkable. Nervous breakdowns occur when the emotions overload and cause the system to crash. Saying "he's too controlling" suggests that it is time to leave, before the matter becomes constricting and volatile.

Teenagers go at "breakneck speed" and tend to hurtle themselves into situations before they think them through, usually because they lack any understanding on how to pace themselves or slow down. This often places them in dangerous situations, such as driving too fast, taking drugs, getting into bad relationships or having early sexual experiences. As the pituitary gland controls the adrenals, the events during the teen years may repeat and extend into adulthood as the lack of caution leads to further bad decisions with regard to jobs, location and type of friends chosen, as they "thrown caution to the wind."

Children living in unstable environments often become emotionally unstable as adults as the emotions encoded in the body at that time, begin to play out in later life. Often labeled rebellious, wild and unpredictable, these people may find that instability from childhood then becomes the norm. Insecurity or abuse of any kind usually leads people to take one of two paths through life, to close down and fail to achieve, or to become a "risk taker"—which is really a cry for help.

> The Greeks knew the pituitary gland as the organ of perception of higher worlds.

The pituitary gland is about being connected to others, in careers and in families, and feeling that the "ground will support us" as we move ahead. If we "see the future" and like what we see then we grow towards it and prosper. If not, we "short ourselves" on opportunities and will never "rise to the occasion." So, will we "go with the flow" or go against it?

Those who exert too much pressure may demand more than we can give, or want to give. Pressure from demanding family members, a boss who expects too much, or a relationship that demands too much time may "push us down" or push us to the edge. But if we feel excited about our own ability to grow, then we will not allow others to "keep us down."

A lack of interest in sex can link to the pituitary gland, as it regulates the sex hormones, estrogen and testosterone. We may "not be in the mood" and not know why and see it as a purely emotional problem, but the emotions work in tandem with the functioning of the body, and once one thing is unbalanced it unbalances other areas too. When the body and emotions work in unison then the "sky's the limit."

See Adrenals, Thyroid, Kidneys, Ovaries and Genitals for additional information.

PROSTATE

Basic Anatomy

The prostate gland is a little larger than a walnut and is situated between the penis and the underside of the bladder, in front of the rectum. Part of the male reproductive system, the gland is small at birth and gradually increases in size throughout adolescence, and sometimes beyond. In a man's late 40's it may start to grow slowly again, increasing the chances of inflammation and prostate problems.

The main function of the prostate gland is to produce and secrete the seminal fluid, which carries spermatozoa. The fluid is milky white in appearance and slightly alkaline in order to neutralize the acidity in the woman's vaginal tract, prolonging the life of the sperm.

During the male climax, the gland is aided by muscles to help propel the liquid into the man's urethra, along with sperm from the testicles, for ejaculation through the tip of the penis. The combined fluids are called semen. Nerve bundles run along the prostate and control the erection, which is why erectile dysfunction often follows prostate surgery. The urethra also runs through the prostate, transporting urine from the bladder to the penis.

The three main health problems connected to the prostate are cancer, an enlarged prostate and prostatitis, which may also be linked to problems with the urinary tract.

Prostate cancer, which grows slowly and usually affects older men, forms in the tissue of the prostate as the cells grow out of control.

An enlarged prostate, called benign prostatic hyperplasia or simply (BPH), affects a large percentage of men and occurs when the cells in the inner core of the gland multiply. As the enlargement puts pressure on the urethra, it causes pain when urinating and a constant feeling that the bladder isn't empty. It can also cause incontinence.

Prostatitis is an inflammation and infection that causes a burning or itching sensation and usually produces a discharge from the penis—and sometimes, also, fever and fatigue.

Emotional disharmony

The prostate is part of the male sex organs and so is connected to how men feels about their sexuality and their place in society. Older men who have prostrate problems or prostate cancer, indicates a faltering of how they feel about aging, not being the "lover" they always imagined themselves to be, and being unable to perform the sex act.

The impotency many men feel in later life can be linked to the status at home or work: losing a job, no longer being a figure of authority, not feeling needed, losing a spouse or loved one, a divorce, or lack of companionship. Prostate cancer is a crisis of faith about being a male in a society where women are making gains, especially in the workplace, as the balance of power is changing. The image most men have of themselves is one that revolves around the genitals and their performance, so a weakening of the penis function leads to a weakening of self-esteem. And as the rules change and anger rises, so the penis deflates.

In our culture, sperm is connected to making babies and being man enough to be able to make them. Men who can't make babies are often seen by other men as lesser beings—which is why, in the past, women were blamed for infertility. "Real men" can perform at the drop of a hat, but not being able to perform is a blemish on manhood. A performance, however, can be the performance at work or at home, and it can reveal how much power is wielded there and who really "wears the pants." Many think of this as the emasculation of men, but in truth, a lot of younger men have moved with the times and share all the responsibilities a family brings. But the increase in prostate cancer today shows how unsure men are of their place in society or in relationships, and unsure if the job they have is still relevant—or in some cases, if they still have a job.

Problems with sexual performance are connected to the end of youth, and an end to attracting women. Male impotence is like female menopause, and are the reason both genders are now turning to plastic surgery to boost self-confidence and to look younger and more appealing to the opposite sex.

Retired men often have prostate problems as they no longer feel useful in society, especially men who invested them-selves in their job and not their home life. Those who haven't prepared for retirement see their lives as having little value, which is why in the past, many men died within a couple of years after retirement.

Prostate problems can affect men at any age, even young men, and because the prostate is linked to the acidity of the vagina, problems can turn into bitterness and resentment at how strong women have become and how relationships have changed. If negative in tone, then a corrosiveness will pervade future sexual relationships. Difficulties can also trace back to some acrimonious situation that caused a sour-ing of a relationship: a bitter divorce or a divorce with high child support payments, a nasty business partnership, older children who have gone their own way and no longer value parental advice, or a sibling rivalry that was never resolved.

For some, the sex act is a game of one-upmanship, one of getting the upper hand over a partner, seeing sex as a one-way street and not playtime for two. Today, many men feel bitter at having to spend money and time on a partner in order to get sex at the end of the evening.

An enlarged prostate will often put pressure on the bladder, causing frequent urination, but pressure can also come from situations at home or work. Pressure to perform better on the job, demanding family obligations, or pressure from money worries, can all affect bladder control and the letting go of the fluid at inopportune times, just as the erection doesn't come at the appropriate moment or doesn't happen at all. Fear of rejection, too, can cause pressure to build especially in older men, but it can also be caused by a need to let a person or situation pass on and to stop hanging on to the bloated negativity.

Words

When women, and other men, want to put a man down, they usually refer to his sexual prowess, which is the way many men prove their manhood to other men. Women can give birth as a mark of their femaleness, while men have to use other things, such as the size and ability of the penis, to produce an equivalent male sense of accomplishment and power. It's the reason some men don't like to look at other naked men in magazines, in films or on television, since comparisons of other men's genitals with their own can undermine their confidence.

Money is equated with power and power with sexual dominance, and a prostate problem may come from lack of money and not the sexual act. We refer to the ability to perform on a job the same way we refer to sexual ability, with sentences such as "he can't get it up," or "he can't perform," or, even worse, "he's not performing at the top of his game." Those who can't perform in any capacity are called "losers," and losers are usually not rich, so rich men are often seen for their sexual prowess as much as their money. Society may condemn their extra marital affairs, but they are frequently applauded by other men.

Many men wonder, "Am I up for the task?" when starting a new job or relationship, or being a father with a second family—all things connected to performance. "I'm not sure of my ability to do this" will often translate into impotency, and if age is a factor, they ask, "Am I too old to be a parent again?" indicating the fear of starting over. We put the words, "act" and "performance" together as if putting on a show, which for many men it is, especially with a younger wife.

> Ronald Reagan didn't become President until he was almost 70 years of age, and during his second term he underwent surgery for an enlarged prostate. Obviously, he was wondering if he was still "up to the job."

Men who are "hen pecked" and constantly berated by a stronger wife, are emasculated, which deprives a man of his male identity. We make jokes about henpecked husbands, but in reality the situation constitutes verbal abuse, just as it is when wives are constantly put down.

Men speak very indirectly, especially about anything personal, so references to prostate problems are often worded as matters of authority, strength and seniority, as they tell others, "I gave him a piece of my mind," in order to look strong. To be "fired from a job" becomes "I think it's time to retire," and "I'm not going to stand for this any longer" also implies that the penis won't stand for it either.

"I don't feel I can do the job any more" may be about work, but in our culture, work is also linked to who we are, how much we are paid, our social standing and our ability and confidence, all of which affect how we are able to function.

We also think of women as being "used," especially in a sexual context, but many men are used by women in order to marry, have a child, or make a spouse pay exorbitant child support. All various ways to "catch" a man. In a "bitter" divorce, when a woman wants to show the husband "who's the boss" and "who wears the pants," she tells her friends that she "got the upper hand." Alternatively, it may be the husband speaking of his wife, but if the resentment becomes "enlarged" and the anger turns inwards, then it may produce prostate cancer, which would indicate a "hollow victory."

See Genitals and Bladder for additional information

SHOULDERS

Basic Anatomy

The shoulder joint is formed by a ball shape at the top of the upper arm bone, called the humerus, which sits in the shallow socket of the shoulder blade (scapula). Three main bones form the shoulder system: the scapula, clavicle and humorous.

The scapula is a flat triangular bone that lies over the back of the upper ribs. It serves as the attachment for muscles, tendons and ligaments that allow for the rotation and upward swing of the arm.

The clavicle, also called the collar bone, is a curved bone that meets the scapula on the top of the shoulder at one end, and the sternum—the breast bone—at the other end to form a strut across the shoulder. It is an important area for muscle attachment connecting the shoulder to the neck.

The humerus, or upper arm bone, inserts into the scapula and together form the glenohumeral joint, which is protected by a bursa, a small sac filled with synovial fluid to protect the rotary cuff. The cuff is a collection of muscles and tendons that surround the glenohumeral joint to give support and motion to the arm and shoulder. The rotary cuff is often the area that sustains an injury and where the tendons of the rotary cuff are torn away from the bone. The muscles and tendons from the shoulder connect the neck, chest, spine and arm.

The ball and socket mechanism, much like that of the thigh, gives a wide range of motion to the upper arm, allowing it to be raised and to rotate. Due to its complexity and high degree of mobility, it is also less stable than other joints. Unlike the hip joint, which actually does fit into a socket, the shoulder joint rests on just a portion of the socket and is held by muscles, tendons and ligaments.

Emotional disharmony

The shoulder connects the arm to the body, allowing it to move freely as it turns, swings, and rotates, but problems with the shoulders indicates our feelings towards that physical freedom and the freedom in the space around us, including the people who are in that space. Do the arms swing easily? Is there a problem turning the arm? Can we put our arms over our heads in a protective way, or raise them towards heaven, as in a religious gesture. If the ball is not rotating well in the socket, then the arm gestures are not rotating well either. Anxiety may be the reason, or doubt regarding our own ability to go after what we seek.

Shoulders that are hunched over can affect anyone at any point and usually connect to depression, grief and tiredness at life. When we feel fine, we lift our head up high and throw back the shoulders, making walking easier and reshaping the whole body into something more relaxed. Shoulders that round and stoop, push the head lower as the body begins to curve and hunch over. Trying to protect ourselves against abuse, verbal or physical, will often pull the chest area inwards, leaving the back and shoulder area to take the abuse. And shoulders that are held high and shorten the neck, indicates stress and fear. Men, especially, have shoulders in this position, which usually comes from formative years spent trying to hide from bullies, unkind words and actions. This is the area where the muscles overlay, making it difficult to release them once they tighten, and if one shoulder is more stressed than the other it can result in back problems. Constantly holding heavy things on one side of the body can also throw off the balance of the neck, shoulders, spine and hips.

Shoulders help carry heavy loads. We carry backpacks strapped onto our shoulders and often hoist children onto them as a way to carry them. Weakness or injury in this area is often a reflection on what's happening in the home or at work. The workload may be too much, due to a boss or coworker piling on assignments, or we may feel that we are being used as a pack horse by family and friends; helping them move furniture, carrying shopping for aging parents, being asked to do tasks that are too time-consuming, or even helping out at school or an organization. If this is the case, then we need to do something to lessen the load, which often requires the word "no," a short word that often seems so difficult to say.

Tightness in the shoulders will hold back arm movement and eventually shorten the muscles down the back, across the chest and in the neck, resulting in pain and an imbalanced body.
A dislocated shoulder occurs when the ball at the top of the upper arm bone pops out of the socket, often tearing the tendons that connect it to the bone. A weakness in this area can be related to a weakness in moving forward and an inability to "carry the load." We can also dislocate the shoulder when we fall and try to catch ourselves, but, since legs and arms are used in movement out into the world, falling shows a faltering belief that we will be all right if we venture out.

Sports and manual labor can produce shoulder problems by pushing the muscles too hard, but the trouble may arise from the feelings we have towards the game played and the job.

Maybe we never wanted to play the sport in question, and we dislike our job intensely. Repetition of the same arm action will also harm the shoulder joints at some point, which is why ball players have trouble.

Problems in a marriage can often result in broken bones, or dislocations, as the marriage is broken in two. If the injury affects the male, it may be seen as a breakdown of the workhorse of the family and reflect resentment at being placed in that position. Or, if we are the one with the injury, it could be that others are splitting apart: parents, siblings, stepparents, partners, and the hurt arm is mirroring the hurt we feel watching the relationship crack. Shoulder trouble may also be a way to gain attention or to bring the two sides back together. We can also "dislocate ourselves" from a marriage or partnership, or from family and friends who may no longer be supportive of the change of direction we wish to take in our job or location. Or that we feel adrift and dislocated from others.

Shoulders that are broken or injured in an accident, can have an emotional component before the event. Falling off a ladder while fixing a home is often about not wanting to fix our own home, or the home of a parent, siblings, ex-wife or another. It may also be that we are leaving the home and really don't want to leave, or that we don't want to leave those who live in the house. The accident is a way to remain together longer. Car accidents usually occur when we are going or coming from some event, situation or meeting that has made us feel weakened. Perhaps we were belittled, chastised, ignored, or we didn't want to attend in the first place.

Inflammation of the shoulder, called bursitis, is caused by internalized anger. It has a burning feeling that makes any action painful, so who or what has caused the anger? If the inflammation recurs, what situation occurred just before the flare-up? If it is a constant pain, then what or who caused the constant irritation: a spouse, parent, coworkers, boss? Is it one particular person, many people, or a situation such as a job, location or lifestyle that is causing distress and anger?

Words

Often, the words we use about a particular part of the body are quite literal, at other times the words describe much more than the indicated area. "Throwing" is a word we connect to the shoulder, but arms, hands and the neck area are also connected to the throwing action. However, when talking of not being able to "throw off a cold" we could also be talking about respiratory problems.

If we want to finish a relationship and to "throw him/her over," we consider it to be finished, but if we are on the receiving end, then we say that "it threw me for a loop" or "it threw me off balance" to describe what a shock it was to receive the information. To throw anything requires a certain amount of strength if we want whatever we throw to land a long way from us. If it's a relationship, then we want the person at a distance. If it's a situation, then we want to distance ourselves from it—usually because we have been hurt, humiliated or upset.

If we are having difficulty with the shoulder, then the ability to throw will be impaired. So who has weakened our ability to "shake off" whatever we wish to be rid of? Someone abusive, a business transaction that has gone sour, a difficult situation at work, a family member who is too clingy, or a needy spouse?

The word "swing" has much the same connotation as "throw" since it requires a healthy shoulder joint in order to swing the arm, If we don't have enough room "to swing a cat" then we feel restricted and not free enough to do the things we'd like to do. Being a "real swinger" suggests someone who is hip, cool and a player. They have enough space, money and charisma to really "play the scene," which is something most people equate with freedom. Not having enough space, money or ability "cramps the style" just as it cramps the movement of the body.

Alberto R. Gonzalez was appointed the U.S. Attorney General in 2005. Called to testify before Congress on issues ranging from the Patriot Act to U.S. Attorney firings, he mostly pleaded ignorance. His neck disappears into his shoulders, so he's not likely to "stick his neck out" on any issue.

We expect men to "shoulder the responsibility," implying that women's shoulders are not sufficiently broad enough to carry the weight. And we give people the "cold shoulder" when we wish to distance ourselves from them or when they have done something offensive. At other times we "shoulder the blame" when we have dome something wrong and are willing to admit it.

The shoulders represent strength, both our resolve and our ability to function well at our job, at running the home and in physical activity. We talk of ourselves, or others, as having "broad shoulders" to shoulder whatever load we have to carry, emotional or physical, and we give others a "shoulder to cry on" when we are feeling strong enough to support ourselves and another.

Decades ago, coal was delivered in bags that were carried across the shoulders of the delivery men to a coal chute which went down to a cellar. They were capable of "carrying the load." Today, many of those same chutes are used for goods delivered to restaurants, while others have been discontinued altogether, just as our muscles, resolve and strength have also weakened due to doing sedentary jobs.

The shoulders are where we carry burdens, willingly or grudgingly, and if the latter, then the load will appear to be heavier as time goes on. But who are we shouldering the burden for, children, spouse, parents, coworkers, friends? Do we feel "put upon" but still remain silent? Are the upper body problems related to feeling stifled by too much responsibility? Are we being "worn down" by an abusive relationship?

The elderly often shuffle, with the body bent over when they don't feel that life has anything more to give them as they speak of "feeling tired and worn out." They have no more strength to carry the burdens of life and are often "spent." But this word is also connected to money, and the exhaustion they feel may be due to a depletion of money and resources.

See Lungs, Arms, Neck for additional information.

SKIN

Basic Anatomy

Weighing approximately 6 pounds and covering the entire surface of the body—about 20 square feet—the skin is the largest organ of the body. It not only functions as a protective barrier against bacteria and infection, but also regulates body temperature, stores water, fat and vitamin D, prevents water loss, and acts as the sense center for pain. It has three main layers: the epidermis, or outer layer, which sheds about every 2 weeks, and the dermis and subcutaneous tissue below.

The characteristics of the skin vary according to which part of the body the skin covers. The head contains more hair follicles that anywhere else, while the soles of the feet contain none. The palms of the hand and soles of the feet have thicker layers, and the eyelids the thinnest layer.

The outer layer, which provides a waterproof barrier, is made up of cells called squamous cells and beneath those are cells called melanocytes, which produce the pigment melanin, giving the skin its color. Both of these layers can develop skin cancer caused by ultraviolet light from too much sun exposure.

The dermis lies below the epidermis and consists mostly of collagen, a protein that gives the skin durability and resistance. The dermis also contains sweat glands to regulate the temperature of the body, as well as hair follicles, and blood and lymph vessels. Sweat and sebum—an oily substance that keeps the skin from drying out—reach the surface of the skin through the pores.

The deeper layer, the subcutaneous tissue, is made of fat, connective tissue, larger blood vessels and nerves. This layer produces lipids, the fatty layer that cushions the inner organs and muscles against damage, and also acts as an insulator against temperature fluctuations.

Emotional disharmony

The entire volume of skin is where the body meets the external world—often a hostile, unkind world, forcing us to become thick-skinned in order to navigate our way through it. As skin covers the entire body, so different areas connect to different emotions, but overall, skin represents what we present to others and how we feel about presenting it. Glowing skin shows our luminosity, while dull, colorless skin reflects our inner dullness, worry and unhappiness. Healthy skin represents a healthy respect for ourselves and confidence in who we are and of what we have to offer.

Unwanted substances such as toxins and pollutants are released through the skin by sweating or by being forced out in the form of a rash or skin eruptions. The irritant may be someone in authority, an annoying situation that just won't go away, or a toxic environment.

The skin also stores fat and water, shown externally in the form of excess weight and edema—a water imbalance in the body that causes swelling, usually in places like the feet. Fluids relate to crying, colds and urinating, all ways to expel unwanted emotions, and are also linked to the kidneys and fear. Unshed tears for a past event, an unresolved childhood trauma, fear of moving into a new job or location, or fear of losing the ability to care for ourselves. Swollen feet represent an inflammation of emotions that make it difficult to walk, so are we in the place we're supposed to be, or in one that feels wrong to us? Are we being asked to move against our will, perhaps to a nursing home or to move in with a family member, or are we too afraid to make the move? Skin swells when something irritates it, such as a sting or an allergy that penetrates below the surface, so what do we want to keep hidden, or who is "getting under the skin" and causing the irritation as our bodies swell in reaction to it?

Skin is the area that we take the most care of, nourishing it with creams and lotions externally, while neglecting the internal areas. But the skin is porous, and not all creams are beneficial, especially those with chemicals in them as they can pass through the barrier of the skin to affect the internal organs, the blood supply and lymphatic system. Reactions occur if we are allergic to certain chemicals in creams, medications, perfumes, foods, or even other people wearing creams and perfumes. A healthy immune system will deal with irritants before they provoke an allergy, but if the allergic reaction recurs, we need to pay attention to where we were just before the reaction took place, or who we were with. Such a reaction is a response to something we have taken in: words, actions, location, environment, liquids or foods. A severe allergic reaction is a small irritant that has become a full-blown negative response.

Dry skin, eczema or psoriasis, is a drying up and a pulling back from social interactions. When our skin is unsightly, we tend to hold back from exposing ourselves to others and stay away from people or important functions and events, leading to missed promotions and other opportunities. Dry skin can affect any area, but often it affects the hands, head, face and arms, which are external, while other times it appears between the toes—movement—and around the groin—intimate and sexual. We may feel exposed and vulnerable in our present situation or be trying to end a relationship, and if itching goes along with the dry skin, then something or someone is causing a constant irritation that we can't disengage from. Itching conveys a desire to scratch away the present situation to get to something new and wanted, a different lifestyle or location, different friends, to move away from family.

Lack of water, which provides fluidity in our movement and shows withdrawal of energy when depleted, can dry up job offers and other prospects. On the other hand, dry people tend to be cynical, emotionless and droll, probably based on past events that have caused them to lose faith in their abilities. We pick at dry skin, just as we pick at others and find fault with everything they do. A picking away at our own layers in the hope that we will uncover our own perfection.

Peeling skin is the shedding of our public image as we move to a new one. We tend to change our appearance when we want something new and exciting, and just as our thought process changes, so the old also has to be peeled back to allow the new to emerge. Peeling skin usually affects the fingers and the feet as we move into new situations and reach out for new experiences. It can also suggest a rolling back of our protective covering as we become more secure and confident.

Cracking skin is the breaking apart of our outer covering, showing vulnerability and allowing bacteria to move in. But the skin also sheds to allow new skin to grow as we move to a better situation, one that will produce a better covering for us in terms of more money, a better locale, or elevated status. The covering can represent housing, or the protection of a partner who has money that will make us feel more protected.

Blisters are a buildup of fluid trying to cushion the flesh beneath. They often appear on the heel from wearing shoes that have rubbed the skin, but they can also be around the mouth and other parts of the body. But is it really the shoes that are ill-fitting, or do we wear them to please others and not ourselves? And what are we trying to protect ourselves from? If the blister is around the mouth, then we are trying to stop others from getting too close or ourselves from saying too much and the blister is a constant reminder to "guard our mouth."

After surgery, we get a scarring of the skin as the area around the cut hardens. It is the way the body protects itself from invaders, and surgery is invasive as the skin is cut purposely. The scarring may be external but the imprint of the surgery is internal, and even though we may never recognize it as such, the scar is there to remind us. The scaring can become much less noticeable as time goes on, but if the emotional upheaval doesn't recede then the scarring won't either. If the surgery was to fix a particular problem but it wasn't successful, then the scarring will also remain—along with the scarred memory that we endured the pain, but got none of the gain.

Words

The skin is our protective covering and shows how protected we feel. It is also an organ that leaves us vulnerable to a hostile world, forcing us to become "thick skinned" as we try to negotiate through the harshness. If we have a negative reaction to others who "get under our skin," or "make our skin crawl" then we know intuitively that something is wrong. The latter feeling is an unpleasant experience, and people who are able to "get under the skin" are usually undesirable, and we should take it as a warning to walk away, even if we lose something in the process. To stay, may place us in danger.

The thinning skin of the elderly is due to its diminishing layer of fat, and reveals the veins more prominently as they return the blood to be re-oxygenate for new life. Thinning skin shows vulnerability, which is perhaps a fear of not getting anything back in return. Having a "cushion against inflation" or something to "cushion us" from the blows of life, such as financial or health problems, gives us a "soft landing." Not having a cushion can mean a harsh outcome is in store.

> Snakes shed their skin as a new one grows, and caterpillars become butterflies so that they can experience more of life by flying—not crawling.

We try to "protect ourselves" from abusive people, but those who verbally abuse know that it shows no visible marks, leaving us with little proof other than the internal bruising. When others talk of needing to protect themselves, they could mean they are in an abusive relationship or have a belittling boss, or that they are trying to protect themselves economically, so do they need help or are they able to handle the situation?

"I jumped out of my skin" implies that something small or large frightened us, and in a relationship where someone gives us one shock after another, affecting our physical and emotional health, then it may be time to leave. Skin shouldn't jump and so putting "jump" and "skin" together implies that maybe we should be the one jumping—away from them—unless we want to "jump for joy."

Skin responds to negative words in the form of a rash, acne, cuts or bruises, and the place where the marks appear will indicate where the weakness lies: face, arms, back, chest, legs or groin. When we are in good health, the arms fight back, the legs run from danger and the groin repels unwanted sexual overtures.

We "sweat" things out when we're hot or want to get rid of something humiliating, or we can "make them sweat" when we turn the tables on others. They can also "rub us the wrong way" to make us angry, although rubbing causes friction that grinds things down eventually, so are we being ground down by circumstances and people or are we the one doing the grinding? If we sweat under the arms or in the groin, the irritation may be sexual, or maybe we are thinking of someone we'd like to "hang out to dry" but can't—a family member, boss, or someone else in authority.

Skin itches when we have a strong reaction to a problem that needs to be scratched away. The problem may be at work or home, so it's important to track when the itching starts and stops—if it does stop. Itching usually happens at certain times and then disappears, so where, when and with whom do we start to itch?

We "peel away the layers" when we try to go deeper into who we are and to answer the question "Why do I keep making the same mistakes?" Delving into the past is part of going deeper into who we are so that we can finally stop peeling back the painful layers from childhood to deal with the anger, sadness, or dissatisfied that we felt at the time.
Perhaps we had a family we were ashamed of, or wished things to be different; parents, siblings, location, school, friends. Now that we are older we can change things, including the voices telling us, "This is the way life is and you can't change it."

We talk of "goose bumps" or say "Someone walked over my grave" when we experience an unwanted sensation. Horror movies often give us this sensation, but so, too, can people. If we hear ourselves saying these words when we see a particular person, we might consider what it is about them that stirs such uncomfortable reactions, and whether it will produce a dangerous situation if we don't remove ourselves. Goosebumps also happen when we are cold, so what does the cold person represent?

Brides on their wedding day are often spoken of as "glowing." "Glowing" people generally have extrovert or spiritual personalities and are willing to open themselves up to others. They often have the ability to shine a light on situations that need to be faced or resolved. Are we glowing or sitting in the shadows? Waiting for others to shine a light or determined to shine our own?

See Cuts, Bruises, Lymphatic system and Cancer for additional information.

SMALL INTESTINE – *Obesity*

Basic Anatomy

The small intestine is 18 to 22 feet long and an about an inch wide and looks like a long, narrow, coiled tube, compacted into the abdominal space. Extending from the stomach to the large intestine, it is divided into three areas, the duodenum, jejunum and ileum, and is responsible for most of the food absorption of the three major classes of nutrients—proteins, fats and carbohydrates.

The first segment, the duodenum, receives the partially digested stomach contents along with pancreatic enzymes and bile from the gallbladder. Food enters the duodenum through the pyloric sphincter, and when enough food has entered it signals the stomach to stop emptying. Peristaltic action—which is a wavelike muscular contraction that moves the food forward—then churns the food together with the enzymes and juices to decrease stomach acidity.

From the duodenum the digested mass passes into the jejunum, where most of the nutrients are absorbed into the bloodstream. The churning action continues and absorption is helped by a vast area of folds, villi and microscopic microvilli, which are thousands of tiny finger-like projections that protrude from the lining of the intestinal wall.

Ultimately, the ileum absorbs most of the the remaining nutrients, especially vitamin B12, bile salts and fluid, before passing the remains into the large intestine. Bile is also absorbed here and returned to the liver through the blood vessels.

Emotional disharmony

It takes about six hours for a meal to pass through the small intestines, and as the brain is linked to the digestive process, so our thoughts will also pass through very slowly too. This is where food breaks down and is sorted before moving into the large intestines for the final processing before it moves out of the body. It is also where our thoughts are broken down too, thoughts about how nourished we feel by the food winding its way through the digestive system, and how nourished we feel in life generally. How enriching the thoughts are can be seen by how well the intestines function.

The digestive system is where we let negative thoughts putrefy if undigested food slows to a crawl, or where it is pushed through too quickly, expelling both food and thoughts before we have had time to digest them. And as the small intestine is connected to the pancreatic duct, it is also where bicarbonate is released in order to neutralize harmful acid coming from the stomach. Acid is corrosive and eats away at the things it comes in contact with, just as we too can become eaten up with bitterness, which if not processed will make us ill-tempered, with an inclination to throw acidic words at others. Unfortunately, the throwing action doesn't always result in a direct hit, so we should be careful when we do feel bitter and resentful at those we lash out at.

Food that gets stuck in the small intestine can come from thoughts and words that we were forced to swallow and that have now passed from the stomach undigested, and any blockage along the way is an inability to allow the emotions to move on freely too. So what words did we hear that upset us? Humiliating words, that have left us with a bitter taste? Angry words that belittled us at work? Annoying words in a family dispute that made us feel unsupported?

Today, digestive disorders are on the increase, but how much of it is connected to lack of good foods, good relationships and a good working environment? We settle for second best instead of demanding something better, something that would feed the mind and the body, and something that would give enough time in the day to digest our foods well. We work long hours that leave little time to enjoy meals with others, and we buy food that is quick to prepare but not nutritious. The result is a host of negative emotions that nag at our digestive system as we move further away from our goals due to a constant barrage of things to take care of, and then slide into eating fast food that gives instant gratification but no long-term relief as we become sick and obese.

We tend to clump the words "obese" and "overweight" together, although, there is a difference, as obesity is a result of body fat as we put on weight, and being overweight can be caused by muscle mass, heavy bones, or fat and water content. We put on weight for different reasons, sometimes to keep us apart from others, sometimes from stress, other times from unhappiness or grief, but it comes from the same thing, feeling unloved or no longer needed. Food can become addictive, especially when it becomes a substitute for love and attention, so we may be slowly killing ourselves from too much food, or from a desire to be perfect.

Obesity may result from having a heavy family where large was considered normal, or from a childhood where there was deprivation, or from just an adoring parent who kept piling on food so that the child was never allowed to encounter a lack. This feeding can also be a form of control by a needy parent wanting acceptance from their child. Accepting the food becomes a form of personal acceptance, too, as the child interprets the weight gain as a sign of love, which then keeps the food coming in order to keep the positive words coming. Eating then becomes an addiction, not to food, but to the reassuring words from someone the child loves. As they see it, if they lose the weight, then they will also lose the love. In some families cooking equates with love and adoration, and not eating much is seen as not appreciating the one who has spent time over a hot stove, which often sets in motion family disputes when food is refused—so better to keep eating!

Obesity can also turn the other way, producing bullies who play out their aggression on those smaller and more vulnerable than themselves in order to detract from their own feelings of vulnerability. It is a cry for some positive words instead of the hurtful words they hear constantly about their weight and size. The overload of weight is a substitute for an overload of negative emotions. In the West we celebrate slim, cute kids and infer that obese kids are somehow not lovable. As the latter get older, for many that image magnifies as their ability to lose weight becomes more difficult and they feel less lovable.

Obesity is also connected to clutter, only this time it's clutter of the body that manifests as external clutter, and as the eating and the weight increase, so the clutter piles mount due to an inability to move easily. It becomes a spiral effect, with the person doing less and less activity but eating more and more—and feeling more and more depressed as the clutter mounts along with the weight.

Many who are obese are really malnourished since they eat food with little nutritional value, but if the mind/body is never satisfied then the constant eating will continue. Changing the diet to a more healthful one, with fewer empty calories, will help the weight loss process as the cravings will decrease and the digestive system will feel satisfied for longer periods of time. Drinking sodas for the sweetness also adds to weight gain, but does little for the sweetness that is really being craved. Losing weight and feeling healthier would help attract more friends and social meetings, which are better conduits for love. Holding on to fat may cushion the blows from the harshness of life, but it will do little to lessen the emotions that are longing for a loving relationship.

Words

The act of processing necessitates that we work through whatever it is that we are dealing with to reach a conclusion. When we say, "I can't process this," the food and the emotions are trying to work through the intestines to reach a conclusion, namely, the end of digestion. We do the same thing when we want to bring closure to a problem, event or relationship that has become difficult. Or perhaps we want to move on and others are the stumbling block, or we may be unable to break down the problem into manageable pieces to delegate, and feel obligated to do all the work ourselves, which is now overwhelming us.

A "gut reaction" is an instinctive response to a situation that requires careful consideration in order to make a decision. Unfortunately, we usually dismiss the gut response, and in the process make the wrong call. A gut reaction is connected to the brain, which is sending a strong message to listen. Problems that we don't have time to fully understand and admit that we "can't digest all this information in time," can produce stress that allows the problem to "get away from us." This is when we need "time out" for ourselves to regenerate so that we can function at a higher level.

The Body's Emotional Imprint

When it comes to being overweight the words used commonly involve denial, like the excuses "I'm big boned" or "I don't eat much." The unspoken truth for many, though, is that although meals might be small, the snacking going on between the meals is very large.

If we are "carrying the load" at work or home, we may believe that we are overloaded and that others are not "pulling their weight." In truth, it could be that the weight is slowing us down and we are the one not pulling the load. Wanting to drop the weight implies a desire to work or be with others, and to be more social.

Weight gain has serious repercussions both in terms of health and in work situations where promotions may be denied because of what the weight suggests to those in charge, such as inability to perform certain tasks. Denial is one way to deal with the problem and talking of wanting to "lighten the load" is another, but denial implies that we won't drop the weight to please others, even if it is doing us harm. Wanting, and stating that we want, to shed the weight implies a desire to look and feel better for ourselves, which involves self-love and how much of it we are willing to give ourselves by slimming down.

> Sigmund Freud proposed that our decision-making and many of our feelings are based on things that we are not really aware of—hence our "gut" feeling.

In relationships, if we no longer want to "carry him around any longer," then we want to leave the relationship and the person who is not doing their part to make it work. But if we are the type of person who volunteers for too many things and takes on too much work and then complain about "carrying the load," then we may be making ourselves sick from an overloaded digestive system that is too sluggish to work well from "eating on the run." An overload can be about money problems, health, family demands, or stress that is impacting our health.

If we really feel "out of sorts" and our digestive system is slow, then we respond to others with irritation. Passing a lot of gas can make people feel unappealing and cranky, which is probably where the derogatory term "gasbag" came from, but gas can also explode, maiming those around—so beware.

See Colon, Stomach, Liver and Skin for additional information

SPINE – Scoliosis

Basic Anatomy

The spine is the backbone, a column of 33 individual bones called vertebrae, that extends from the neck down to the pelvis. These vertebrae, which stack one on top of the other, have a gelatinous filled cartilage disk between each one to cushion and absorb shocks and to allow for motion. This column also gives structure and support to the spinal cord. A bundle of nerves that extends from the base of the brain to the lower back and is the nerve center for the entire body, transmitting messages that facilitate movement to the torso, head and limbs. It is divided into four areas; the cervical, thoracic, lumbar and sacral.

The spinal cord feeds through the spinal canal—small openings in the vertebrae through which the spinal cord runs—and has 31 pairs of nerves that are responsible for transmitting messages from body to brain and back again in order to control bodily functions. Shorter than the actual spinal column, the spinal cord ends before the sacrum vertebrae.

The cervical vertebrae start at the base of the skull with seven bones; the nerves in this section are responsible for most of the movement from the shoulders up. If the nerves of the cervical spinal cord are badly crushed or damaged, organ failure, lack of mobility and paralysis may result.

The thoracic, middle section of the spine, consisting of twelve vertebrae, are responsible for most of the nerve action from the waist to the shoulders, especially the internal organs.

The lumbar section, the five largest vertebrae in the column, are used for lifting, bending and supporting the body's weight. The spinal cord nerves from the lumbar region down, work the internal organs and the lower limbs.

The final section, the sacral, located at the base of the spine, consists of one triangular shaped bone called the sacrum that connects the spine to the pelvis. In a child, it is made up of five separate bones, but by the teen years they fuse into just one.

At the very end of the spine is the coccyx (tailbone), four bones formed into one, that give protection and support when sitting. Connecting the entire vertebral column together are two long, thick ligaments that run the entire length of the spinal column, with smaller ones between the vertebrae.

Emotional disharmony

The spinal column is the powerhouse for the entire body, as it keeps us upright and allows us to bend, stretch and perform tasks. This is where we hold our convictions about who we are and whether or not we are willing to become part of the backbone of society. It is about freedom—to move, to participate, to take action. The spinal cord is the nerve center for all of our actions and so wherever problems exist in the spine, they also correspond to the emotional aspects of that area too.

The upper portions of the spine represents the shoulders, neck, head, face and the brain—and being alive. A hump in the middle of the back at the neck, often referred to as a dowager's hump as it usually affects older women, is the holding back of anger and resentment and being unable to voice those emotions.

The middle section denotes an inability to grasp for the things we want as it relates to the functioning of the lungs, heart, liver, kidneys and digestive systems. We may be able to move towards our goals, but we need the good health of the organs to get us there.

The lower and middle back is the place that takes most of the strain when we haul heavy objects. If we have back problems, we usually blame ourselves for not lifting something the right way, but emotionally the problems can relate to what we are being asked to lift. We may resent moving boxes into or out of a new home, or doing the action for others. Or the move can be because of a job loss, divorce, or moving away from parents who have had enough of a slacker kid. Lifting heavy objects for a living and feeling tired of the job and seeing no end in sight and no way to move on, can produce debilitating back problems. We may not be able to take the action to leave the job, but the strained back muscles can force the action.

Back problems related to the lower portion of the spine, involves difficulty with the legs and pelvis—including the bladder and reproductive organs—and indicates an inability to move forward and to feel centered and strong enough to perform the action.

Scoliosis shows conflict and is congealed energy that causes the muscles to contract, limiting them from extending to their full capacity, which can occur after a trauma or emotional event, or during some ongoing family misery. It is the armoring of the upper part of the body as we try to protect ourselves from verbal or physical blows, or see a loved one experience abuse while we feel incapable of protecting them. Thoughts are encased in the muscles, and distortions occur according to which side is pushing and which side is pulling:

the mother or the father, the bully or the subservient person, wanting to go but needing to stay. And as the two sides battle it out, we try to become smaller by compacting the spine in order to stay out of harm's way. Divorced parents may have put us in a difficult situation where we are expected to take sides, or parents who argue and have placed us in the middle of the battle, forcing us to duck down in order to avoid the arrows that are flying.

The fact that scoliosis occurs in children and teens, at their most vulnerable time, is very telling as it shows the relationship between the home environment and the external one.

Most curvatures are towards the top of the spine and affects the ribcage, indicating that the problem has to do with having a voice, reaching out for what we want, being able to breathe freely and feeling loved in a safe, nurturing environment.

It's important to remember that bones don't move themselves, or become distorted on their own: something has to pull or push them, and that's the job of the muscles. Any distortion of the skeletal structure is caused by the way the muscles tighten or relax; if the bone structure is distorted, then the muscles have pulled them down, much like a young tree blown by a constant wind that causes it to bend and then remain in that position. Trees and plants do the same thing as they strain towards light, curving and changing to reach sunlight, even if just a sliver of sunlight is visible.

Conflict can also result from not liking what the body represents, especially as we usually like one side more than the other—and prefer to show our "better side" to others. Feeling more vulnerable on one side of the body than the other comes from how secure we feel being male or female.

The Body's Emotional Imprint

Back problems originate from too much responsibility or from too many demands, and as the spine is responsible for so many actions, so the emotional range plays out too. Feeling responsible for family members, carrying problems at work or with a spouse, or moving into a new relationship or marriage, often requires that we carry a heavy load which is sometimes beyond our capacity. At other times we overload ourselves by not delegating or asking others to pull their weight: families who don't clear up after themselves, siblings who won't share the burden of an aging parent, a spouse who wants all the perks but none of the work.

As we age, the cushions between the vertebrae decrease in size as the spine shrinks accordingly. But the shrinking can come at any age if we feel that we have lost our status as a strong provider or feel that we are no longer relevant at home or work. Back problems can also arise from trying to stand up for others who are weaker, testing our own strength and resolve.

Words
Words connected to the spine usually refer to how strong, secure and centered we feel about the direction we are going in. "I'm not sure about anything anymore" is said in response to having to make decisions for the future, but we are really speaking of the break down of the support system that was supposed to help us to get where we wanted to go. We talk of not "feeling supported" when those who were supposed to support us, don't: a spouse, parent or family member we thought we could count on. If our resolve falters in the face of mounting resistance, our backbone will falter too.

Today, as the underpinnings of society are collapsing and our health is suffering along with the collapse of nature, the words about lack of support are more evident. The economic system of countries, as well as the food and water supply, are all failing, which in turn makes us feel insecure and "unsupported." We feel alone and adrift in society, and as jobs become less certain, so those who are working often have to support their families on one income instead of two.

The spine is the support system for our entire being, and so phrases like "I feel as if I'm carrying the weight of the world" and "Life is just too much for me" are signs of our structure's fatigue as it starts to cave in. But who is making us carry the load and do we really need to carry it? Is there a way to share it, or are we not good at delegating? Often we only see solutions through our own eyes, leading to a one-sided solution, so which side is taking the load?

> While moving boxes into his new home, after leaving the White House, Dick Cheney pulled a muscle in his back. He was in a wheelchair when he attended the 2009 presidential inauguration. Obviously, he wasn't going to stand for any man!

Many phrases we say are related to feeling overloaded, just as we would feel if we were carrying a very heavy load on our backs. But even though we say "My back aches," we are really stating that emotionally we can't carry the load any longer. The ache may be in the back but it can also relate to an overloaded nervous system that is struggling to keep up with too many messages from too many sources—just as we as a society are also struggling with an overload of messages from too many sources.

Words that form spinal distortions or back problems are often produced by the words we speak to ourselves, words that we repeat like a mantra. "I hate my body." "I wish I wasn't here." "I wish I looked like that," are all ideas which, if uttered enough times, will take its cue to make the body overweight, less tall, and less of a target. Sometimes the words "I couldn't think straight" seem to fit other physical parts of the anatomy, but if the spine is curving then what upset if causing the emotions to become unbalanced and out of alignment?

When directed at others, the words "I'm sick of trying to straighten out his/her life" or "I can't support all his nonsense any more," take their toll as we become the caretaker and assume responsibility for others, eventually constricting our own life as the vertebrae are compressed down and we are left alone to "iron out all the kinks." Carrying the load for those who refuse to do their fair share can sometimes force us to shout, "Get off my back!" In society there are those who are very responsible and those who are not, and the latter are usually good at "shifting the load" to the responsible ones who are unable to let things slide. Ask those less responsible, though, and they say that they see no great need to "carry the load." So is it a load that really needs to be carried? Or is the need to be responsible left over from childhood, when we were chided for "not pulling our weight?"

On the other hand, the word "rub" has good and bad connotations as we can rub someone's back for pleasure, or "rub people the wrong way." The action of rubbing can produce friction, so where is the discord from, a spouse, boss, coworker, partner, parent, sibling? Is there an end to the friction or will it continue to be unresolved, wearing away the one who feels that they are being "rubbed the wrong way" and forced to "back down." If it leads to emotional pressure, it may be time to walk away from the situation. No job or relationship is worth losing our health for.

"Spineless" people who have "no backbone" are perceived as weak, but it could be their situation that is making them weak, such an abusive relationship, or a situation at home where they are given more responsibility than they can cope with, or they may simply be silent about their situation as they deal with elderly parents, an alcoholic spouse, or money worries.

This perception of weakness could also refer to the fact that the spine really is compacting down, so who is saying the words, us or others? On the other hand, bones become brittle and inflexible when they don't have enough calcium, and that can result from drinking too much coffee and soft drinks which draw calcium out of the bones in order to provide more to the blood supply. If this happens for long enough, the bones will become brittle, causing other problems around the compacted spine. It can also cause the words to become brittle and harsh when directed at others.

See areas that correspond to the spinal sections for additional information.

SPLEEN

Basic Anatomy

The spleen is a soft, purplish organ about the size of a fist and lies just under the left side of the rib cage next to the stomach. Weighing between 5 to 7 ounces, it serves as a reservoir for blood in case of emergencies. Part of the lymphatic system, and the largest single organ in the immune system, its function is to fight infection, keep the body fluids in balance and help control the amount of blood in the body. Humans can survive without a spleen but will have a greater risk of infections.

The spleen's main function is as a filter for the blood, removing toxins and infecting organisms, and to remove old and damaged red and white blood cells and platelets—which help blood to clot—while allowing healthy blood cells to pass into the bloodstream for circulation. Cells that are unable to pass through have their iron extracted and are then returned to the bone marrow where the cells are destroyed by lymphocytes, a type of white blood cell.

An enlarged spleen (splenomegaly), occurs when it has to work excessively to manufacture or filter the blood cells and platelets, reducing the number of healthy cells in the bloodstream. It can also result from viral, parasitic or bacterial infections, and liver disease or cancer.

Emotional disharmony

The spleen is a true warrior organ in that it repels invaders, cleans out the unwanted and recycles the old. And just as it fights with infections, pushes out toxins, clears outworn blood cells from the bloodstream and balances fluids, so it does the same thing emotionally. When working well, the spleen brings stability to the system as it balances force with practicality so that one doesn't over rule the other, just as the ability to deal with the old and the new requires the facility to make way for the new, but also to utilize the old when necessary. If the system backs up, however, then stagnation will occur, leaving the emotions to do the same as they turn into irritability, sourness and anger.

Balancing requires an even distribution of something in order to make it fair, steady and equal, whether it's balancing planks of wood, a check book or emotions. Are we willing to work with others, or are we resentful of having to work within a unit when we would rather be working on our own? Are we working for someone else when we'd rather own our own business? Are we in a relationship we'd rather walk away from? Do we have to do a balancing act to hold a team together, either at home or at work, while others gain the rewards?. Doing all the work but never getting the recognition eventually builds up anger and resentment, which then alienates others and stops us from working harmoniously.

Unlike the lymphatic system, which runs through the entire body, the spleen is localized on the left side, the female side, and not standing up for ourselves is often considered a female trait. Sometimes we allow resentment to accumulate by holding on to grudges and hostilities from past events, which, if we are unable to release them, will affect our ability to fight off people and infections, and leave us vulnerable to invaders and those who will do us harm. Is a situation harming us physically or emotionally, and if so, who is involved? Or are we harming ourselves by not asking for help? If we are in a toxic situation or with toxic people who take pleasure in bringing us down, then it's essential to remove either them, or ourselves.

Sometimes the words that we say about others can also apply to how we live. Accumulating clutter is the same as collecting too much unwanted emotional baggage, and living with clutter is often about living with the past, with something that should be dead and buried, something, or someone, who should have been cleared out a long time ago.

The spleen is where we hold worry, usually irrational worry about things that may never occur: lack of money and how protected we feel, or about others who could do us harm. If we feel unable to fight back and hold our own in a marriage, family or work-related situation, we may worry about the possible consequences. Perhaps about how to protect children from a violent or unhappy marriage, or from an overbearing sibling intent on having their way in a family dispute. Is the worry real or unfounded? Can a solution be found? Have we become the voice of reason in the family and ended up performing a balancing act between two warring factors?

An enlarged spleen reflects an enlargement of the entire emotional situation, which has been allowed to grow out of control and beyond its borders, an event that was not been dealt with in a timely fashion, or, when there was an opportunity to do so. When we feel bloated, we become irritable and lash out at others as our feelings drag us down and makes us feel tired, out of sorts, apathetic and "stuck."

Words
We "vent our spleen" when we are apoplectic at someone and believe we have been taken advantage of or unjustly treated and now feel the need to spew out our anger, although,

we can also vent at those who are not the intended target. Our words usually signify that we are not able to fight back or that life is "draining away" as the strength to fight back is weakened. Anger that increases to "seeing red," the color of blood, shows the need to go after someone's "blood" so that we can release our anger and move on. The spleen, if working well, will cleanse the blood and clear out all the old, worn or damaged cells, just as we often do with people in our own lives.

The spleen seems to inspire writers. William Shakespeare describes the irritability of a character in Julius Caesar as "You shall digest the venom of your spleen." Jane Austen wrote "Adieu to disappointment and spleen." And Alexandre Dumas was more emphatic, "there is nothing more galling to angry people than the coolness of those on whom they wish to vent their spleen."

When we talk of others having a "toxic energy," we mean that they are "poisonous" to be around and pose a danger to our emotional state—just as the accumulation of anything toxic is a danger to those around it. Toxins that can't be released are destructive and if taken internally can make us sick. Any kind of weakness makes us less able to fight those who wish to bring us down, whether it's in a work environment or another situation where they have the upper hand. Walking away from the situation—and finding a new job or relationship—is probably better than expending the energy to stay and fight, since some things, or people, are just not worth the emotional distress.

Resentment also builds when people refuse to release others from their grasp, or on the other side, those who are caught by others blocking the way; parents who won't allow their children to leave emotionally, a divorced spouse who refuses

The Body's Emotional Imprint

to believe that the marriage is over, a business venture that has gone sour. As the anger and frustration build, we often "vent" at whoever happens to be in the way, usually at an inopportune moment. Unfortunately, the one with the health problem is usually the one trying to leave, not the one blocking the way.

If we constantly feel "beaten down" or "stuck in the job" or "weary and despondent," we need the help of others to free ourselves from the situation that is "bringing us down"—before the situation really does bring down our health. On the other hand, if we express the wish to "get rid of all the clutter," this is a positive goal that requires a positive action to match, even if it requires hiring someone to help in the action. "Getting rid of the old" can be positive and bring a move to a new place, a new job, or a new relationship—and a better life. But hanging on to outworn situations or people can drag us down to be unproductive and hostile.

Alternatively, people who are "full blooded" tend to be adventurous, lively and in demand socially. We talk of a "real full blooded man/women" as one who is fun-loving, energetic, hearty, with stamina to finish the course, and who possesses everything else a man/woman could want of a playmate.

See Stomach and Lymphatic system for additional information.

STOMACH - Food Allergies

Basic Anatomy

The stomach is a hollow, curved, muscular pouch about 10 inches long that sits to the left side of the chest. Connected to the esophagus at one end—the tube leading down from the throat, and the duodenum at the other—the first part of the small intestine, its main job is to help process food and store it until required by the small intestines, enabling us to eat two to three meals a day instead of eating continually. The initial part of the digestive process is triggered by sight, smell and taste.

The esophagus runs behind the windpipe and in front of the spine and is the tube that allows food to pass from the mouth to the stomach, where it is broken down by digestive juices containing enzymes and hydrochloric acid (HCL)—an acid that kills many harmful organisms in food.

Ridges of muscle tissue, called rugae, line the stomach walls and contract when the stomach is empty and then expand as food is consumed. Moving the food along are muscles that contract periodically to help digest the food with a churning motion. The average adult stomach can expand to accommodate around 3-4 liters of food, which usually remains in the stomach for two to four hours after a meal.

Between the stomach and the duodenum is the pylorus, a long narrow passage surrounded by a thick ring of muscle called the pyloric sphincter, which regulates the passage of chyme—a semifluid mass of partially digested food—as it passes to the duodenum.

Although much of the food breakdown occurs in the stomach, the entire digestive process starts in alimentary canal—a tubular passage that extends from the mouth, through the esophagus to the stomach, then to the small intestines and colon, to end at the anus. In an adult, the entire canal can be about 27 feet long.

An allergic reaction to food—often a reaction to an entire food group—can be hereditary, but more often it results from the immune system perceiving something in the food as harmful. As a way to protect the body, the immune system produces antibodies and releases them into the bloodstream. One of these chemicals is histamine, which produces allergy symptoms that may affect the eyes, nose, throat, lungs or skin, and as the antibodies recognize the offending food each time it is eaten, it releases the histamine, initiating the allergic reaction.

This reaction, often severe, will usually occur within a couple of hours after eating, sometimes within minutes, and it can be mild or severe causing symptoms that include abdominal pain, diarrhea, difficulty swallowing, swelling of the eyes and face, and itching of the mouth. Food intolerance is often mistaken for an allergy, but intolerance doesn't involve the immune system, even though some of the symptoms may mirror those of an allergy.

Emotional disharmony

The stomach is were our intuition/gut reaction dwells and where we feel nurtured or neglected, and since in our society food equals love, feeling unloved usually pushes us towards foods that are nutritionally depleted and unhealthy. Eating such foods infers that we don't feel worthy of anything better, although in our culture it is seen as an act of self-love when no one else is willing to love us.

Depleted foods are exhausted foods that have lost most of their nutrients, and eating them will also make us feel depleted and without energy, leading to depression, listlessness and a feeling of being gorged. Who have we allowed to deplete us of vitality and the joy of life? A money problem or a situation that is draining us emotionally? A boss or coworker who makes us feel sick to our stomach every time we walk in to work? A family member who never has a good word to say to us? A past relationship that just won't move on emotionally?

As part of the digestive system, the stomach is responsible for breaking down the food and storing it until it is released into the small intestines. Hydrochloric acid is one of the gastric juices in the stomach that helps protect us from bacteria and also aids in the digestive process, but too much of it can cause a burning sensation called heartburn, which results when the acid has backed up into the esophagus and produced a sour, bitter taste.

Acid is destructive and corrosive, as it can burn through the hardest of metals, and when related to the digestive process can produce people who are acidic in tone and sour towards others. It can also produce feelings of despondency and melancholy as we turn on ourselves for things we've done or should have done, not accomplishing as much as we'd hoped, or our parents had hoped, or making bad decisions with bad results, in marriage, relationships, business transactions.

If we constantly have heartburn, then we have allowed something to back up in our life that should have been moved on, and the very name "heartburn" indicates that the problem is connected to the heart and love—or anger. Who or what situation is making us turn on ourselves and what changes can we make to turn things back again. Are we yearning for a lost love, or bitter about a broken marriage and a costly divorce?

If the problem is an over acidic body, then eating more alkaline foods can bring the body—along with the emotions—back into balance, and enzyme supplements will also help rebalance it. Or, for a quick fix, a half a teaspoon of baking soda in a glass of water is fast acting.

Feeling bloated can be relieved by chewing gum for a few minutes right after a meal—gum produces saliva that activates the digestive juices and moves the food along faster.

Food represents mother, love and everything that a secure home symbolizes, all the warm, cuddly things that remind us of childhood, and feeding the belly is a substitute for that mother love. Our foods today have less nutritional value than a few years ago, due mostly to agribusiness never letting the soil replenish itself, which in turn is producing a malnourished society. Similarly, we feel starved of love in life and relationships, with too many things to do, too much to take care of, too much of everything, except the things that would nourish the body and soul. The need to snack constantly is an indication that we are not being nourished at meal times, but much of that comes from eating "empty calories," which fill us for a while but then leave us feeling hungry again before the next meal arrives. This is the treadmill effect: we try to lose weight but then eat snack foods that are fattening in order to fill the void.

Today, many are allergic to foods such as wheat, dairy, nuts and gluten, and the list keeps growing. But what are we really allergic to and is it really an allergy or a reaction to something, someone, some situation? Allergies can appear at certain times in our lives and then disappear, especially when connected to stress. Getting married before we are ready for the responsibility, feeling overwhelmed in a recurring situation, family demands, or feeling stress at work can bring on reactions that can play out in different parts of the body—eyes, nose, skin, mouth, lungs, stomach. Often, when the cause of the emotional upset is dealt with, the allergic reaction also clears up.

Being hypersensitive to foods means that we are also hypersensitive to situations that cause allergic reactions. Carbohydrates equate with sweetness, bulk, fullness, and the solidness of the things we need to support us, but emotionally, the allergy translates into a feeling that life is no longer full, or sweet, or satisfying.

Today many are allergic to gluten, found mainly in wheat and other grains. But gluten is the glue that binds things together, the stickiness that forms dough to make bread. In the past people had a family unit to support them, but today many no longer feel supported, not by the government, religions, family or friends, many of whom are also feeling overwhelmed and unsupported themselves. Women are the glue that holds most families together, and they are feeling under siege, which coincides with the fact that women are more likely to be gluten-intolerant than men. Many feel alienated, let down and unsupported in marriages, jobs, or pregnancy, with too many family obligations and too much stress in business.

Protein builds strong muscles and bones and is found in many foods: meat, dairy products, nuts, legumes and seafood—all foods we have consumed throughout the ages. A protein allergy is to feel weakened physically and emotionally and represents being in a situation where others are in a stronger position; a relationship with an overbearing spouse, boss, or

The Body's Emotional Imprint

family unit. Milk also represents mother's milk and nourishment, and today, women are still fighting to be allowed to breastfeed their babies in public, and just as our bones are weakening, so is the whole social and infrastructure.

Indigestion is caused by something that can't be digested, including undigested emotions that have not been assimilated and absorbed, often because of family friction at meal times: eating with parents who ask too many questions; eating with a spouse or partner we are afraid of; eating where there is underlying tension, where anger is always part of the meal. Children are often the ones impacted by family upheavals, and the stomach is usually the first place affected.

Ulcers, often called peptic ulcers, are sores that develop on the inside lining of the stomach, the small intestine or the esophagus; they are an irritation that has grown enough to cause abdominal pain. Many believe that bacteria is the cause, but bacteria can only take hold if there is a way to enter, such as a weakened immune system. Stress and acidic foods can exacerbate the problem, and stress is often caused by not addressing a situation in a timely manner which then allows the ulcers to grow. This can be a "sore point" about money, a problem in a relationship, or something that is wearing us down as we become sore at others. A family squabble over money that is causing a hole to develop within the family unit? A condition that is eating away at the unit or burning up the money? An unresolved problem that is growing into something much bigger?

Words

The stomach is where we digest reality, or at least our interpretation of reality, and if we have stomach problems and feel "sick to our stomach," then the reality is crushing us. So what reality is making us sick and allergic? Kids have stomach aches when they are asked to do things they feel nervous about, such as standing in front of the class, or playing sports, or when they feel unable to deal with a personal situation such as dealing with a bully at school. Any situation that makes us feel "I can't stomach this" is one which we feel unable to face or solve.

If we are "sick of the place," then the actual location, or the people there, or type of work we do at that location, may actually be making us sick. The air quality could be unhealthy, the work environment not conducive to workers getting along, or the commute too long. Or it could be a marriage that is over, or a home that never feels like home, which usually connects back to an unhappy childhood that we now experienced in our adult home. We don't always see the link between situations from childhood that have traveled with us, and the problems we encounter as adults.

In 1992 near the end of a trip to Japan to drum up U.S. trade, President George Bush, while attending a formal dinner, vomited over the Prime Minister of Japan. The inference was plain.

If we tell ourselves, "I'm not in a good place right now," the actual place may indeed be bad for our health. We may not understand what the problem is, but these words imply that something is affecting us and we should pay attention. Is the place dangerous and so makes us feel unsafe? Are people verbally abusive? Or are we feeling constricted by where we are living?

Sickness in the stomach often shows a fear about doing something that is wrong and knowing that it is wrong, causing the body to vomit anything from the stomach in order to get rid of the distasteful thoughts. Bulimics consume a great amount of food in a short time and then stick their fingers down the throat, or use laxatives, in order to purge the meal. Their reason is often an abnormal body image of themselves, which translates into a distancing of anything or anyone who could nourish them in a relationship. Many are involved in professions where image is important, and being perfect is expected.

When we vomit, we release hydrochloric acid, a harsh chemical that can eventually eat away at the stomach, esophagus, throat and the enamel on the teeth. The throat is where we have a voice, where we state our opinions; it is also where we swallow, often, words we wish we could say. And since many more women are bulimic than men, it is also about society "eating away" the autonomy of women and women feeling unable to fight back.

Wanting to throw-up on a continual basis, as many bulimics do, shows a desire to mutilate the body from the inside and deprive themselves of anything that would make them healthy and attractive. It is also a cry to stop others from being critical and eroding their self-esteem and by constantly making them feel worthless and unlovable.

Often, we talk of others "bugging us" when we want to be alone. But bugs burrow and so getting "bugged" or catching a "stomach bug" refers to a situation that is like a bug that never leaves the body. They get "under the skin" and "eat away" at us, just as we have allowed others to eat away at our self-defenses.

See Gall Bladder, Throat, Teeth for additional information.

THYROID GLAND

Basic Anatomy

The thyroid is an important part of the endocrine gland, which release hormones into general circulation. Shaped like a butterfly and weighing less than one ounce, it is divided into two lobes that wrap around the front of the windpipe (trachea). The thyroid hormone is essential for every cell in the body, for it regulates metabolism. Thyroid cells are the only cells in the body that absorb iodine, a trace mineral found in many foods, and converts it into hormones that are released into the blood stream to be transported throughout the body. This process regulates metabolism—converting food into energy—and also helps regulate the heart, blood pressure and body temperature.

The thyroid is controlled by the pituitary gland, a small pea-size gland situated at the base of the brain, which stimulates the thyroid into producing more hormones when levels fall too low.

Two main thyroid problems, which are usually more common in women, arise when there is either an overactive thyroid—hyperthyroidism—or an under active thyroid—hypothyroidism. Hyperthyroidism is caused by the overproduction of thyroid hormone, which can cause an increased heart rate, weight loss, fatigue, anxiety, difficulty sleeping, muscle weakness, greater sensitivity to heat, irritability, and even infertility. Hypothyroidism is caused by the underproduction of thyroid hormone, and can cause weight gain, fatigue, depression, greater sensitivity to cold, dry skin and hair, constipation, difficulty thinking clearly and poor hearing.

Although these problems are usually connected to the thyroid, they may also be caused by the pituitary gland.

Emotional disharmony

The thyroid gland, small though it is, is responsible for the functioning of so much, including our growth, metabolic rate—energy required to keep the body functioning when at rest—and for temperature control. The metabolic rate is also related to weight gain and weight loss, and keeps the body balanced, not too hot and not too cold, which in turn keeps our emotions balanced as we endeavor to grow physically and spiritually. It is the balance between who we are and who we wish to become, between thought and action.

The small gland wraps around the trachea, the passageway between the head and the body that allows air to pass from the nose and mouth down to the lungs, so any blockage here will impede the air flow and cause us to gasp for air. Words that cannot pass through, will also get stuck as they wrap around the thyroid, obstructing the movement of the words, and people with thyroid problems very often are in relationships where they have little voice. The partner may be overbearing, controlling and "always right," and so even if there is dialogue, it will probably be a one-way street. When we breathe freely, oxygen can circulate around the body and enables us to speak our mind, something that many women are not allowed to do, or think they should not do.

The adrenals and thyroid are both parts of the endocrine system and are closely linked. The adrenals regulate adrenaline and cortisol production for the fight-or-flight response, while the thyroid regulates hot and cold temperatures, so both glands deal with balance. Do we, or others, blow hot and cold? Do we have a boss who is calm and stable one minute but flies off the handle the next, or do we live with a spouse who has constant mood swings, or with parents or siblings who argue incessantly. All of which, can cause stress to the one who is left to do the balancing act and play referee.

Any upset with the thyroid can produce fatigue, hair loss, dry skin, depression, weight loss or gain and a host of other problems, which are often misdiagnoses as concerns of other areas of the body. Many of the emotional symptoms mirror adrenal problems, such as fear, stress and a difficulty in being able to balance life, relationships or work loads.

The gland is like the furnace of a building, heating it to a required temperature and then turning off for a while, but if it doesn't turn off then it will produce too much heat. Hyper, as the name suggests, refers to an overactive thyroid that produces too much heat, causing an increase in perspiration, sleepiness, rapid heartbeat and muscle weakness, while hypo is a low-functioning thyroid that makes the person sensitive to cold and can produce infertility, depression and brain fog.

Women tend to be affected with thyroid problem more than men, which may account for weight fluctuations and constant tiredness, but which could also be attributed to carrying the load at home and at work, and by skimping on good nutritious meals at mealtimes.

Words
When we talk of life being "out of balance," it may well be our health that is out of balance and we are draining ourselves dry by constantly running from one thing to another without taking the time to replenish ourselves. If this phrase refers to a sensitivity to heat or cold, and our emotions are

"blowing hot and cold" with others, then the thyroid may be unable to find any "middle ground." Feeling too hot tends to slow us down, making every action an effort, and feeling too cold can make us miserable and snap at others.

Growing anything requires attention and support from others, but it also requires that we have enough room to "have our say" about whatever is being grown. We may have high hopes and dreams, but will remain silent if others choose to "dampen the fire" or "rain on our parade." The words of optimism are there, but are being choked by others who are cold and unresponsive. Or, we may be in a relationship where the partner/spouse leaves us feeling cold and physically drained as their needs overriding our own.

As the thyroid regulates the rate at which the body burns energy, so it also helps to control our weight. An increase in weight can make us feel "sluggish" and "slow," while those who "eat like a horse"

George Bush suffered from Graves' disease—an overactive thyroid—during the first Gulf War, and many questioned whether that had any bearing on his decision to go to war. Once diagnosed and given medication, however, he slowed down to the point that many questioned whether his uninspired second term presidential campaign was due to his medication.

and find it difficult to increase their weight, may be slowly wearing themselves out. Weight can also represent an emotional load that is dragging us down, and, since the thyroid is located between the head and the body, the problem can also be a clash between what we want to do versus what we think we should do. As one side pulls against the other, it can seem as if we are "at war" with ourselves, which usually means that everything and everyone around us will also suffer the consequences.

Brain fog leaves us feeling spacey, confused and tired, and with an inability to concentrate. If we state, "I can't wrap my head around this problem" when confronted with a task that is beyond our understanding, we should question whether it is the problem that needs solving or the body that needs more carbohydrates, or thyroxin – an iodine-containing hormone secreted by the thyroid. Alzheimer's disease is also associated with brain fog, and as it usually affects the elderly, it may really be linked to a lack of vitamins, minerals, nutritious food, or enough fluids—all of which can affect the workings of the brain. A slowing down of the brain can make it difficult to go shopping and cook nutritious meals, which will, over time, lead to greater health problems.

Often people on diets see sugar as the enemy and then deprive themselves of the glucose needed to keep the body furnace going. Whole grains and pasta are often the first things cut, but the body needs a "balanced" diet in order to maintain emotional equilibrium, and cutting out the sweet part of a diet can lead to cranky, irritable people who "take it out" on others and alienate those who are needed, leading the dieters back to eating more wrong foods in order to feel loved.

The thyroid is attached to the trachea, and so talk of being "unattached" or "I'm finding it difficult to connect" may be a lack of iodine, which the body cannot make on its own but which is needed in order for the thyroid to function well. Seafood, seaweed and sea salt are rich in iodine and provide the small amount needed to stay healthy. But just as we have to rely on external sources for an iodine supply, so we also have to rely on others for companionship. A thyroid that is

The Body's Emotional Imprint

out-of-balance will lead to unbalanced emotions, which can cause difficult relationships as we alternate between pushing away those we need and clinging to others who may not be able to help us.

As an iodine deficiency produces low thyroid hormones, it can lead to menstruating problems and infertility, and the "cooling" of a relationship, especially if a couple is trying to become pregnant. And if a partner complains that "we're just not close any more" or that the marriage "is cooling," then pay attention. Not feeling "in the mood" may mean that the relationship really is cooling.

See Pituitary Gland, Neck and Adrenals for additional information.

WRIST

Basic Anatomy

The wrist is made up of eight small bones arranged in two rows, known as the carpals. One row connects to the radius and ulna, the bones in the forearm, while the other row connects to the palm of the hand. Covering the meeting point of the bones is cartilage, which cushions the joints and allows the surfaces to slide one against the other without causing damage.

Ligaments, fibrous, connective tissue that bonds bone to bone, surround the carpal bones by a way of a joint capsule which contains a lubricating fluid called the synovial fluid. There are many different ligaments in the wrist area that add strength and support as they connect the bones in the hand, but injury from stretching or tearing can take a long time to heal.

Muscles, which are connected to bones by tendons, cross through the wrist as they travel from the forearm down to the hand and fingers, while the three main nerves that serve the hand—the ulnar, radial and median—pass down the full length of the arm. These nerves cross the wrist and carry signals from the brain to the muscles that move the arm, hand, fingers and thumb, and then carry signals back to the brain about pain, temperature and other sensations.

Running through the wrist is the carpal tunnel, a narrow passageway which encases the nerves and tendons and connects the arm to the hand. Carpal tunnel syndrome, a painful progressive condition, occurs as the medial nerve, which runs into the palm of the hand and controls sensations to the thumb and the first three fingers, becomes compressed or squeezed at the wrist. The constant pressure on the under wrist area, usually from overuse or a repetitive action, can cause tingling, pain and weakness in the hand, or in severe cases, numbness traveling up the arm. Changing work duties to something less repetitive or wearing a splint will often solve the problem.

Emotional disharmony

The wrist gives the hand freedom to change direction as it moves up, down and around and also indicates how we feel about our own ability to change direction. Are we able to move freely, or is there a stiffness in how far we can go? Are we willing to adapt to accommodate others, and how flexible are we willing to be?

The arm and the hand may be willing, but if the wrist isn't strong enough to support the hand movement forward or to grasp for what we want, then movement will be difficult. Aches and pains at this point indicate that there is something or someone blocking the way that is causing us emotional pain too. It may be a job where we have been held back while others have moved forward, or a family situation where someone else is getting the attention.

The wrist may weaken or break when a son or daughter marry and the new spouse takes the place of the parent and becomes a stronger force. The aging parent now becomes less important to their child, breaking the bond that held the family together. Is the injury on the left or right side? Is a daughter leaving or a son? Is there a problem with the son/daughter-in-law who is driving a wedge between the parent and child, just as the wrist has weakened between the hand and the arm. Or is someone at work causing us to break from a situation or project we really want to continue?

Weak bones indicate a weak body structure, and for the elderly a fall often precedes a meeting or a situation where they feel unsupported by family or others who question their ability to support themselves and live alone. A fall often shows that the hand wants to hold on and the arm wants to stretch out to stop the fall, but the wrist is too weak for either action, forcing a break or strain between the two.

A sprained wrist is energy that has become blocked and so blocks us as we strain to reach for what we want, or to reach out to others who could help, or even to put out our hand to ask for help. Problems with the wrist can also bring others into our lives to do the things we are now unable to do—or resent having to do—including a spouse who didn't pull their weight, coworkers who now have to do a little more work instead of leaving us to do it, kids who now have to help out. If children sprain their wrist, then it may be a fear of participating in some sport or activity. Or are anxious about being asked to do something they feel is beyond their capability. They may want to do it, but are hesitant to get involved.

Carpal tunnel is inflexibility in the wrist from typing on computers or doing another repetitive action for too long, leading to an inability to move the hand or the fingers. It usually happens when we have a dislike or fear of computers, or dislike the reason we are using the computer—maybe being asked to do work we begrudge. It could be computer work for an aging parent who can no longer perform the task, or for an organization that we feel is taking advantage of us, or a business that we no longer wish to work for.

If we sit at a desk job all day but hate the work, then developing carpal tunnel syndrome will force us to find a different job. We may not have the courage to stop what we are doing,

The Body's Emotional Imprint

but the injury will make the decision for us. Factory workers and others who perform repetitive motions with the hands and wrist, can all suffer from the same resentment—maybe towards a boss or business—and see no way out of the working environment.

Lack of flexibility will also impede our movement forward, usually in jobs, if we refuse to "bend" to the wishes of others. This can lead to resentment and bitterness, especially in business where others are promoted ahead of us. But our own inflexibility is probably the reason we are constantly passed over.

Emotions connected to the wrist show how adaptable we can be to turn things around quickly, whether it's a product, project, business or relationship—and to do it willingly.

Words

As we age the bones become more brittle and the wrist is where we break a fall, often breaking the wrist in the process. A break of the wrist is to break the hand from the arm. The arm may be willing, but the desire to grasp what is before us, isn't. When we talk of someone as "a very brittle person," it suggests they are hard on the surface and seem to be in control, but who may really be feeling vulnerable on the inside. The word "brittle" suggests something that shatters into pieces when dropped, which is the way many elderly people feel in later life, and having a fall usually shatters their already small world into even smaller fragments. They may fear that if they do shatter, no one will be able to put them back together again and that life as they know it will be over.

Brittle things are hard to the touch, but shatter once dropped. Brittle people have to be handled with care as they can "snap" easily, and often do at others, but they can also snap by falling to pieces emotionally. And just as we take great care of glassware, so we should also be careful with breakable people. These are the ones who alienate others but are really in need of friendship and kindness, which due to their inability to bend a little to accommodate others, can be difficult to give. We say they are unable to "bend even a little" or "refuse to adapt" in order to accommodate those around them, but the inability to work with others may actually relate to real pain caused by stiffness and inflammation, which could account for their inflammatory words.

Falling suggests a vulnerable state, but the words can indicate that they are on the edge and without the support of a safety net. We can break a wrist at any age, so it important to see what preceded the fall, or what ongoing situation weakened the ability to stop the fall. Money problems may be the cause, or a support that has collapsed, such as the death of a loved one. The situation can also force others to "pick up the pace" and relieve the pressure. Or it can show the injured that they are not indispensable and need to delegate more.

> The wrist is the bridge point between the potential of the arm, and the inclination of the hand to fulfill it.

If we complain that others have "twisted my words," it usually indicates that they needed to to make themselves look better to someone in authority. These are insecure people who should be avoided, and if they just receive a "slap on the wrist" for their meddling, then the best recourse is to "take the high road." Negative emotions usually affect the offended party far more than the guilty one, so if the unfairness continues move to a different job, spouse or location—one where truth is appreciated.

Carpal tunnel syndrome results from stress across the nerves that lead into the hand and can cause a numbing or painful sensation. Feeling "numb" or having a "bad feeling" about a direction taken, is a sign that a situation isn't being addressed and that the hand is being deployed in the wrong area, such as not taking care of the "business at hand," which has now stopped the money from flowing through. Billing and accounting are the nerve center of any business, and the "numbness" may be the numbing of reality to the financial problems. Paying someone to work on the computer and do the accounting will often alleviate the wrist problem, along with the financial one.

See Arm and Hand for additional information.

Author's notes

The writing of this book actually began many years ago, as I was seeking more information on alternative health, but became sidetracked when I started an organizing business called "Tame the Space." Seeing the connection between the piles of clutter and certain emotional patterns, and understanding that clutter forms in the mind long before the hoarding begins, I wrote the book *The Emotional Imprint of Clutter.*

Most of us find our way to natural health in order to address our own health problems, and I was no exception, but the emotional aspect always intrigued me, too. My fascination with the internal workings of the mind started in high school, when I bought a book by Carl Jung. The following year I fell in love with the human form when I entered Art College and spent ten weeks, 9am to 9pm, drawing the undraped figure. It was a wonderful introduction to both art and who we are externally.

Over the years, I've come to a better understanding of the link between what our bodies are telling us about health issues, and the words and sayings we use to strengthen that message. I discovered that link for myself, when, during a particularly trying time in my life, I experienced muscle weakness in the legs and found myself thinking "I don't have a leg to stand on." Now that the muscles are much stronger, I no longer think of that phrase.

My quest for information about natural health continued over the years as I became certified as an Iridologist—diagnosis by examination of the iris of the eye—and attended many other classes on health-related subjects, including anatomy, which is the reason for including the Basic Anatomy section in this book. The section is a no-frills version with very little terminology as I believe that for the average layperson—me included—the medical terms tend to confuse the issue. All I want to know is "What does it do?"

My thanks, however, to Kathleen Higgins RN, for the time she put into this section, reading and rereading my revisions. I know it was difficult for her to come down to my level, and I thank her for both her patience and imput, although, any mistakes are purely my own.

Those who are already familiar with anatomy will obviously skip this section, but having just a tiny amount of information on the structure and function of the organs and the muscular and skeletal system will help make the emotional connection easier to understand.

The purpose of this book is to show a different way of looking at health issues, and the words and saying I've chosen are just a few that could have been used. You may, and probably will, find many more words that apply to your circumstances.

My sincere thanks, also, to Diana Bloom, who also edited *The Emotional Imprint of Clutter*, for her excellent editing—pulling together my often disjointed sentences—although, again, any mistakes are mine.

Thanks also go to Jim Bisakowski, yet again, for his book designing prowess.

Seeking good health can be both fulfilling and rewarding. May your journey be as interesting as mine has been.

www.ingramcontent.com/pod-product-compliance
Lightning Source LLC
Chambersburg PA
CBHW062046270326
41931CB00013B/2963